MedicalCenter.com

I0422543

The Key Facts

On Cancer Risk Factors

and Causes

The Key Facts on Cancer: Volume III

Everything You Need to Know About Cancer Risk Factors and Causes

-Usable Medical Information for the Patient-

By Patrick W. Nee

www.MedicalCenter.com

Published by:

MedicalCenter.com

96 Walter Street/ Suite 200

Boston, MA 02131, USA

Tel: 617-354-7722

www.MedicalCenter.com

manager@medicalcenter.com

The Key Facts on Cancer Series

Volume I: The Key Facts on Cancer Treatment

Volume II: The Key Facts on Cancer Types

Volume III: The Key Facts on Cancer Risk Factors
and Causes

Volume IV: The Key Facts on Cancer Prevention

Volume V: The Key Facts on Cancer Detection
and Diagnosis

Volume VI: The Key Facts on Coping With
Cancer & Cancer Resources

Table of Contents

Chapter 1: Introduction

What is Cancer?

Cancer is a term used for diseases in which abnormal cells divide without control and are able to invade other tissues. Cancer cells can spread to other parts of the body through the blood and lymph systems.

Cancer is not just one disease but many diseases. There are more than 100 different types of cancer. Most cancers are named for the organ or type of cell in which they start - for example, cancer that begins in the colon is called colon cancer; cancer that begins in melanocytes of the skin is called melanoma.

Cancer types can be grouped into broader categories. The main categories of cancer include:

- *Carcinoma*- cancer that begins in the skin or in tissues that line or cover internal organs. There are a number of subtypes of carcinoma, including adenocarcinoma, basal cell carcinoma,squamous cell carcinoma, and transitional cell carcinoma.
- *Sarcoma* - cancer that begins in bone, cartilage, fat, muscle, blood vessels, or other connective or supportive tissue.

- *Leukemia* - cancer that starts in blood-forming tissue such as the bone marrow and causes large numbers of abnormal blood cells to be produced and enter the blood.
- *Lymphoma and myeloma* - cancers that begin in the cells of the immune system.
- *Central nervous system cancers* - cancers that begin in the tissues of the brain and spinal cord.

Origins of Cancer

All cancers begin in cells, the body's basic unit of life. To understand cancer, it's helpful to know what happens when normal cells become cancer cells.

The body is made up of many types of cells. These cells grow and divide in a controlled way to produce more cells as they are needed to keep the body healthy. When cells become old or damaged, they die and are replaced with new cells.

However, sometimes this orderly process goes wrong. The genetic material (DNA) of a cell can become damaged or changed, producing mutations that affect normal cell growth and division. When this happens, cells do not die when they should and new cells form when the body does not need them. The extra cells may form a mass of tissue called a tumor.

Not all tumors are cancerous; tumors can be benign or malignant.

- *Benign tumors* aren't cancerous. They can often be removed, and, in most cases, they do not come back. Cells in benign tumors do not spread to other parts of the body.
- *Malignant tumors* are cancerous. Cells in these tumors can invade nearby tissues and spread to other parts of the body. The spread of cancer from one part of the body to another is called metastasis.

Some cancers do not form tumors. For example, leukemia is a cancer of the bone marrow and blood.

Cancer Statistics

A report from the nation's leading cancer organizations shows that rates of death in the United States from all cancers for men and women continued to fall between 2005 and 2009, the most recent reporting period available. Estimated new cases and deaths from cancer in the United States in 2013:

- *New cases*: 1,660,290 (does not include nonmelanoma skin cancers)
- *Deaths*: 580,350

The risk of developing many types of cancer can be reduced by practicing healthy lifestyle habits, such as eating a healthy diet, getting regular exercise, and not smoking. Also, the sooner a cancer is found and treatment begins, the better the chances are that the treatment will be successful.

Chapter 2: "Light" Cigarettes and Cancer Risk

- On June 22, 2010, a law that bans tobacco manufacturers from using the terms "light," "low," or "mild" in tobacco product labeling went into effect. However, some manufacturers are using color-coded packaging (such as gold or silver packaging) on previously marketed products and selling them to consumers who may continue to believe that these cigarettes are not as harmful as other cigarettes.

- When tar is measured with a smoking machine, the smoke from a so-called light cigarette has a lower yield of tar than smoke from a regular cigarette. However, people don't smoke cigarettes like a machine, so they may still get a high yield of tar with a light cigarette.

- Light cigarettes are no safer than regular cigarettes. The only way to reduce the risk of smoking-related diseases is to stop smoking completely.

What is a so-called light cigarette?

Tobacco manufacturers have been redesigning cigarettes since the 1950s. Certain redesigned cigarettes with the following features were marketed as "light" cigarettes:

- Cellulose acetate filters (to trap tar).
- Highly porous cigarette paper (to allow toxic chemicals to escape).
- Ventilation holes in the filter tip (to dilute smoke with air).
- Different blends of tobacco.

When analyzed by a smoking machine, the smoke from a so-called light cigarette has a lower yield of tar than the smoke from a regular cigarette. However, a machine cannot predict how much tar a smoker inhales. Also, studies have shown that changes in cigarette design have not lowered the risk of disease caused by cigarettes.

On June 22, 2009, President Barack Obama signed into law the Family Smoking Prevention and Tobacco Control Act, which granted the U.S. Food and Drug Administration the authority to regulate tobacco products. One provision of the new law bans tobacco manufacturers from using the terms "light," "low," and "mild" in product labeling and advertisements. This provision went into effect on June 22,

2010. However, some tobacco manufacturers are using color-coded packaging (such as gold or silver packaging) on previously marketed products and selling them to consumers who may continue to believe that these cigarettes are not as harmful as other cigarettes.

Are light cigarettes less hazardous than regular cigarettes?

No. Many smokers chose so-called low-tar, mild, light, or ultralight cigarettes because they thought these cigarettes would expose them to less tar and would be less harmful to their health than regular or full-flavor cigarettes. However, light cigarettes are no safer than regular cigarettes. Tar exposure from a light cigarette can be just as high as that from a regular cigarette if the smoker takes long, deep, or frequent puffs. The bottom line is that light cigarettes do not reduce the health risks of smoking.

Moreover, there is no such thing as a safe cigarette. The only guaranteed way to reduce the risk to your health, as well as the risk to others, is to stop smoking completely. Because all tobacco products are harmful and cause cancer, the use of these products is strongly discouraged. There is no safe level of tobacco use. People who use any type of tobacco product should quit.

Do light cigarettes cause cancer?

Yes. People who smoke any kind of cigarette are at much greater risk of lung cancer than people who do not smoke. Smoking harms nearly every organ of the body and diminishes a person's overall health.

People who switched to light cigarettes from regular cigarettes are likely to have inhaled the same amount of toxic chemicals, and they remain at high risk of developing smoking-related cancers and other disease. Smoking causes cancers of the lung, esophagus, larynx (voice box), mouth, throat, kidney, bladder, pancreas, stomach, and cervix, as well as acute myeloid leukemia.

Regardless of their age, smokers can substantially reduce their risk of disease, including cancer, by quitting.

Chapter 3: Second Hand Smoke and Cancer

- Secondhand smoke (also called environmental tobacco smoke, involuntary smoke, and passive smoke) is the smoke given off by a burning tobacco product and the smoke exhaled by a smoker.
- At least 69 chemicals in secondhand smoke are known to cause cancer.
- Secondhand smoke causes lung cancer in nonsmokers.
- Secondhand smoke has also been associated with heart disease in adults and sudden infant death syndrome, ear infections, and asthma attacks in children.
- There is no safe level of exposure to secondhand smoke.

What is secondhand smoke?

Secondhand smoke (also called environmental tobacco smoke, involuntary smoke, and passive smoke) is the combination of "sidestream" smoke (the smoke given off by a burning tobacco product) and "mainstream" smoke (the smoke exhaled by a smoker).

People can be exposed to secondhand smoke in homes, cars, the workplace, and public places, such as bars, restaurants, and recreational settings. In the United States, the source of most secondhand smoke is from cigarettes, followed by pipes, cigars, and other tobacco products.

The amount of smoke created by a tobacco product depends on the amount of tobacco available for burning. The amount of secondhand smoke emitted by smoking one large cigar is similar to that emitted by smoking an entire pack of cigarettes.

How is secondhand smoke exposure measured?

Secondhand smoke exposure can be measured by testing indoor air for nicotine or other chemicals in tobacco smoke. Exposure to secondhand smoke can also be tested by measuring the level of cotinine (a by-product of the breakdown of nicotine) in a nonsmoker's blood, saliva, or urine. Nicotine, cotinine, carbon monoxide, and other smoke-related chemicals have been found in the body fluids of nonsmokers exposed to secondhand smoke.

Does secondhand smoke contain harmful chemicals?

Yes. Among the more than 7,000 chemicals that have been identified in secondhand tobacco smoke, at least 250 are known to be harmful, for example, hydrogen cyanide, carbon monoxide, and ammonia.

At least 69 of the toxic chemicals in secondhand tobacco smoke cause cancer. These include the following:

- Arsenic
- Benzene
- Beryllium (a toxic metal)
- 1,3–Butadiene (a hazardous gas)
- Cadmium
- Chromium (a metallic element)
- Ethylene oxide
- Nickel (a metallic element)
- Polonium-210 (a radioactive chemical element)
- Vinyl chloride

Other toxic chemicals in secondhand smoke are suspected to cause cancer, including:

- Formaldehyde
- Benzo[α]pyrene
- Toluene

Many factors affect which chemicals are found in secondhand smoke, such as the type of tobacco, the chemicals added to the tobacco, the way the tobacco product is smoked, and, for cigarettes and cigars, the material in which the tobacco is wrapped.

Does exposure to secondhand smoke cause cancer?

Yes. The U.S. Environmental Protection Agency, the U.S. National Toxicology Program, the U.S. Surgeon General, and the International Agency for Research on Cancer have all classified secondhand smoke as a known human carcinogen (a cancer-causing agent).

Inhaling secondhand smoke causes lung cancer in nonsmoking adults. Approximately 3,000 lung cancer deaths occur each year among adult nonsmokers in the United States as a result of exposure to secondhand smoke. The U.S. Surgeon General estimates that living with a smoker increases a nonsmoker's chances of developing lung cancer by 20 to 30 percent.

Some research also suggests that secondhand smoke may increase the risk of breast cancer, nasal sinus cavity cancer, and nasopharyngeal cancer in adults and the risk of leukemia, lymphoma, and brain tumors in children.

Additional research is needed to learn whether a link exists between secondhand smoke exposure and these cancers.

What are the other health effects of exposure to secondhand smoke?

Secondhand smoke is associated with disease and premature death in nonsmoking adults and children. Exposure to secondhand smoke irritates the airways and has immediate harmful effects on a person's heart and blood vessels. It may increase the risk of heart disease by an estimated 25 to 30 percent . In the United States, secondhand smoke is thought to cause about 46,000 heart disease deaths each year. There may also be a link between exposure to secondhand smoke and the risk of stroke and hardening of the arteries; however, additional research is needed to confirm this link.

Children exposed to secondhand smoke are at increased risk of sudden infant death syndrome, ear infections, colds, pneumonia, bronchitis, and more severe asthma. Being exposed to secondhand smoke slows the growth of children's lungs and can cause them to cough, wheeze, and feel breathless.

Chapter 4: Smokeless Tobacco and Cancer

- Smokeless tobacco is tobacco that is not burned. Smokeless tobacco is also known as chewing tobacco, oral tobacco, spit or spitting tobacco, dip, chew, and snuff/snus.
- Smokeless tobacco causes cancer and other diseases.
- Smokeless tobacco is not a safe substitute for cigarettes.

What is smokeless tobacco?

Smokeless tobacco is tobacco that is not burned. It is also known as chewing tobacco, oral tobacco, spit or spitting tobacco, dip, chew, and snuff. Most people chew or suck (dip) the tobacco in their mouth and spit out the tobacco juices that build up, although "spitless" smokeless tobacco has also been developed. Nicotine in the tobacco is absorbed through the lining of the mouth.

People in many regions and countries, including North America, northern Europe, India and other Asian countries, and parts of Africa, have a long history of using smokeless tobacco products.

There are two main types of smokeless tobacco:

- Chewing tobacco, which is available as loose leaves, plugs (bricks), or twists of rope. A piece of tobacco is placed between the cheek and lower lip, typically toward the back of the mouth. It is either chewed or held in place. Saliva is spit or swallowed.

- Snuff, which is finely cut or powdered tobacco. It may be sold in different scents and flavors. It is packaged moist or dry; most American snuff is moist. It is available loose, in dissolvable lozenges or strips, or in small pouches similar to tea bags. The user places a pinch or pouch of moist snuff between the cheek and gums or behind the upper or lower lip. Another name for moist snuff is snus (pronounced "snoose"). Some people inhale dry snuff into the nose.

Are there harmful chemicals in smokeless tobacco?

Yes. There is no safe form of tobacco. At least 28 chemicals in smokeless tobacco have been found to cause cancer. The most harmful chemicals in smokeless tobacco are tobacco-specific nitrosamines, which are formed during the growing, curing, fermenting, and aging of tobacco. The level of tobacco-specific nitrosamines varies by product. Scientists have found that the nitrosamine level is directly related to the risk of cancer.

In addition to a variety of nitrosamines, other cancer-causing substances in smokeless tobacco include polonium–210 (a radioactive element found in tobacco fertilizer) and polynuclear aromatic hydrocarbons (also known as polycyclic aromatic hydrocarbons).

Does smokeless tobacco cause cancer?

Yes. Smokeless tobacco causes oral cancer, esophageal cancer, and pancreatic cancer.

Does smokeless tobacco cause other diseases?

Yes. Using smokeless tobacco may also cause heart disease, gum disease, and oral lesions other than cancer, such as leukoplakia (precancerous white patches in the mouth).

Is using smokeless tobacco less hazardous than smoking cigarettes?

Because all tobacco products are harmful and cause cancer, the use of all of these products should be strongly discouraged. There is no safe level of tobacco use. People who use any type of tobacco product should be urged to quit.

As long ago as 1986, the advisory committee to the Surgeon General concluded that the use of smokeless tobacco "is not a safe substitute for smoking cigarettes. It can cause cancer and a number of noncancerous oral conditions and can lead to nicotine addiction and dependence". Furthermore, a panel of experts convened by the National Institutes of Health (NIH) in 2006 stated that the "range of risks, including nicotine addiction, from smokeless tobacco products may vary extensively because of differing levels of nicotine, carcinogens, and other toxins in different products".

Chapter 5: Cigar Smoking and Cancer

- Cigar smoke, like cigarette smoke, contains toxic and cancer-causing chemicals that are harmful to both smokers and nonsmokers.

- There is no safe tobacco product, and there is no safe level of exposure to tobacco smoke.

- The more you smoke, the greater your risk of disease.

- Cigar smoking causes oral cavity cancers (cancers of the lip, tongue, mouth, and throat) and cancers of the larynx (voice box), esophagus, and lung.

- All cigar and cigarette smokers, whether or not they inhale, directly expose their lips, mouth, tongue, throat, and larynx to tobacco smoke and its toxic and cancer-causing chemicals.

How are cigars different from cigarettes?

Cigarettes usually differ from cigars in size and in the type of tobacco used. Moreover, in contrast with cigarette smoke, cigar smoke is often not inhaled.

The main features of these tobacco products are:

- *Cigarettes*: Cigarettes are uniform in size and contain less than 1 gram of tobacco each. U.S. cigarettes are made from different blends of tobaccos, which are never fermented, and they are wrapped with paper. Most U.S. cigarettes take less than 10 minutes to smoke.
- *Cigars*: Most cigars are composed primarily of a single type of tobacco (air-cured and fermented), and they have a tobacco wrapper. They can vary in size and shape and contain between 1 gram and 20 grams of tobacco. Three cigar sizes are sold in the United States:
  - <u>Large cigars</u> can measure more than 7 inches in length, and they typically contain between 5 and 20 grams of tobacco. Some premium cigars contain the tobacco equivalent of an entire pack of cigarettes. Large cigars can take between 1 and 2 hours to smoke.
  - <u>Cigarillos</u> are a type of smaller cigar. They are a little bigger than little cigars and cigarettes and contain about 3 grams of tobacco.

o Little cigars are the same size and shape as cigarettes, are often packaged like cigarettes (20 little cigars in a package), and contain about 1 gram of tobacco. Also, unlike large cigars, some little cigars have a filter, which makes it seem they are designed to be smoked like cigarettes (that is, for the smoke to be inhaled).

Are there harmful chemicals in cigar smoke?

Yes. Cigar smoke, like cigarette smoke, contains toxic and cancer-causing chemicals that are harmful to both smokers and nonsmokers. Cigar smoke is possibly more toxic than cigarette smoke. Cigar smoke has:

- *A higher level of cancer-causing substances*: During the fermentation process for cigar tobacco, high concentrations of cancer-causing nitrosamines are produced. These compounds are released when a cigar is smoked. Nitrosamines are found at higher levels in cigar smoke than in cigarette smoke.

- *More tar*: For every gram of tobacco smoked, there is more cancer-causing tar in cigars than in cigarettes.
- *A higher level of toxins*: Cigar wrappers are less porous than cigarette wrappers. The nonporous cigar wrapper makes the burning of cigar tobacco less complete than the burning of cigarette tobacco. As a result, cigar smoke has higher concentrations of toxins than cigarette smoke.

Furthermore, the larger size of most cigars (more tobacco) and longer smoking time result in higher exposure to many toxic substances (including carbon monoxide, hydrocarbons, ammonia, cadmium, and other substances). Cigar smoke can be a major source of indoor air pollution. There is no safe level of exposure to tobacco smoke. If you want to reduce the health risk to yourself and others, stop smoking.

Do cigars cause cancer and other diseases?

Yes. Cigar smoking causes cancer of the oral cavity, larynx, esophagus, and lung. It may also cause cancer of the pancreas. Moreover, daily cigar smokers, particularly those who inhale, are at increased risk for developing heart disease and other types of lung disease. Regular cigar smokers and cigarette smokers have similar levels of risk for oral cavity and esophageal cancers. The more you smoke, the greater the risk of disease.

What if I don't inhale the cigar smoke?

Unlike nearly all cigarette smokers, most cigar smokers do not inhale. Although cigar smokers have lower rates of lung cancer, coronary heart disease, and lung disease than cigarette smokers, they have higher rates of these diseases than those who do not smoke cigars.

All cigar and cigarette smokers, whether or not they inhale, directly expose their lips, mouth, tongue, throat, and larynx to smoke and its toxic and cancer-causing chemicals. In addition, when saliva containing the chemicals in tobacco smoke is swallowed, the esophagus is exposed to carcinogens. These exposures probably account for the similar oral and esophageal cancer risks seen among cigar smokers and cigarette smokers.

Are cigars less hazardous than cigarettes?

Because all tobacco products are harmful and cause cancer, the use of these products is strongly discouraged. There is no safe level of tobacco use. People who use any type of tobacco product should be encouraged to quit.

Do nicotine replacement products help cigar smokers to quit?

Nicotine replacement products, or nicotine replacement therapy (NRT), deliver measured doses of nicotine into the body, which helps to relieve the cravings and withdrawal symptoms often felt by people trying to quit smoking. Strong and consistent evidence shows that NRT can help people quit smoking cigarettes. Limited research has been completed to determine the usefulness of NRT for people who smoke cigars. For help with quitting cigar smoking, ask your doctor or pharmacist about NRT, as well as about individual or group counseling, telephone quitlines, or other methods.

Chapter 6: Harms of Smoking and Health Benefits of Quitting

- Tobacco smoke is harmful to smokers and nonsmokers.

- Cigarette smoking causes many types of cancer, including cancers of the lung, esophagus, larynx (voice box), mouth, throat, kidney, bladder, pancreas, stomach, and cervix, as well as acute myeloid leukemia.

- Quitting smoking reduces the health risks caused by exposure to tobacco smoke.

What are some of the health problems caused by smoking?

Smoking harms nearly every organ of the body and diminishes a person's overall health. Millions of Americans have health problems caused by smoking.

Smoking is a leading cause of cancer and death from cancer. It causes cancers of the lung, esophagus, larynx, mouth, throat, kidney, bladder, pancreas, stomach, and cervix, as well as acute myeloid leukemia.

Smoking also causes heart disease, stroke, aortic aneurysm (a balloon-like bulge in an artery in the chest), chronic obstructive pulmonary disease (COPD) (chronic bronchitis and emphysema), asthma, hip fractures, and cataracts. Smokers are at higher risk of developing pneumonia and other airway infections.

A pregnant smoker is at higher risk of having her baby born too early and with an abnormally low birth weight. A woman who smokes during or after pregnancy increases her infant's risk of death from Sudden Infant Death Syndrome (SIDS). Men who smoke are at greater risk of erectile dysfunction.

Cigarette smoking and exposure to tobacco smoke cause more than 440,000 premature deaths each year in the United States. Of these premature deaths, about 40 percent are from cancer, 35 percent are from heart disease and stroke, and 25 percent are from lung disease. Smoking is the leading cause of premature, preventable death in this country.

Regardless of their age, smokers can substantially reduce their risk of disease, including cancer, by quitting.

What are the immediate benefits of quitting smoking?

The immediate health benefits of quitting smoking are substantial:

- Heart rate and blood pressure, which are abnormally high while smoking, begin to return to normal.
- Within a few hours, the level of carbon monoxide in the blood begins to decline. (Carbon monoxide reduces the blood's ability to carry oxygen.)
- Within a few weeks, people who quit smoking have improved circulation, produce less phlegm, and don't cough or wheeze as often.
- Within several months of quitting, people can expect substantial improvements in lung function.
- In addition, people who quit smoking will have an improved sense of smell, and food will taste better.

What are the long-term benefits of quitting smoking?

Quitting smoking reduces the risk of cancer and other diseases, such as heart disease and COPD, caused by smoking.

People who quit smoking, regardless of their age, are less likely than those who continue to smoke to die from smoking-related illness:

- *Quitting at age 30*: Studies have shown that smokers who quit at about age 30 reduce their chance of dying prematurely from smoking-related diseases by more than 90 percent.

- *Quitting at age 50*: People who quit at about age 50 reduce their risk of dying prematurely by 50 percent compared with those who continue to smoke.

- *Quitting at age 60*: Even people who quit at about age 60 or older live longer than those who continue to smoke.

Does quitting smoking lower the risk of cancer?

Yes. Quitting smoking reduces the risk of developing and dying from cancer. However, it takes a number of years after quitting for the risk of cancer to start to decline. This benefit increases the longer a person remains smoke free. The risk of premature death and the chance of developing cancer from smoking cigarettes depend on many factors, including the number of years a person smokes, the number of cigarettes he or she smokes per day, the age at which he or she began smoking, and whether or not he or she was already ill at the time of quitting. For people who have already developed cancer, quitting smoking reduces the risk of developing a second cancer.

Should someone already diagnosed with cancer bother to quit smoking?

Yes. There are many reasons that people diagnosed with cancer should quit smoking. For those having surgery, chemotherapy, or other treatments, quitting smoking helps improve the body's ability to heal and respond to therapy. It also lowers the risk of pneumonia and respiratory failure. Moreover, quitting smoking may lower the risk of the cancer returning or a second cancer developing.

Chapter 7: Breast Cancer Risk in American Women

- Based on current breast cancer incidence rates, experts estimate that about one out of every eight women born today will be diagnosed with breast cancer at some time during her life.

- The strongest risk factor for breast cancer is age. A woman's risk of developing this disease increases as she gets older.

- Other factors can also increase a woman's risk of developing breast cancer, including inherited changes in certain genes, a personal or family history of breast cancer, having dense breasts, beginning to menstruate before age 12, starting menopause after age 55, having a first full-term pregnancy after age 30, never having been pregnant, obesity after menopause, and alcohol use.

What is the average American woman's risk of developing breast cancer during her lifetime?

Based on current incidence rates, 12.4 percent of women born in the United States today will develop breast cancer at some time during their lives. This estimate, from the most recent SEER Cancer Statistics Review (a report published annually by the National Cancer Institute's Surveillance, Epidemiology, and End Results [SEER] Program), is based on breast cancer statistics for the years 2007 through 2009.

This estimate means that, if the current incidence rate stays the same, a woman born today has about a 1 in 8 chance of being diagnosed with breast cancer at some time during her life. On the other hand, the chance that she will never have breast cancer is 87.6 percent, or about 7 in 8.

In the 1970s, the lifetime risk of being diagnosed with breast cancer in the United States was just under 10 percent (or about 1 in 10).

The last five annual SEER reports show the following estimates of lifetime risk of breast cancer, all very close to a lifetime risk of 1 in 8:

- 12.7 percent for 2001 through 2003
- 12.3 percent for 2002 through 2004
- 12.0 percent for 2003 through 2005
- 12.1 percent for 2004 through 2006
- 12.4 percent for 2005 through 2007

SEER statisticians expect some variability from year to year. Slight changes, such as the ones observed over the last 5 years, may be explained by a variety of factors, including minor changes in risk factor levels in the population, slight changes in breast cancer screening rates, or just random variability inherent in the data.

What is the average American woman's risk of being diagnosed with breast cancer at different ages?

Many women are more interested in the risk of being diagnosed with breast cancer at specific ages or over specific time periods than in the risk of being diagnosed at some point during their lifetime. Estimates by decade of life are also less affected by changes in incidence and mortality rates than longer-term estimates. The SEER report estimates the risk of developing breast cancer in 10-year age intervals. According to the current report, the risk that a woman will be diagnosed with breast cancer during the next 10 years, starting at the following ages, is as follows:

Age 30	0.44 percent (or 1 in 227)
Age 40	1.47 percent (or 1 in 68)

Age 50	2.38 percent (or 1 in 42)
Age 60	3.56 percent (or 1 in 28)
Age 70	3.82 percent (or 1 in 26)

These probabilities are averages for the whole population. An individual woman's breast cancer risk may be higher or lower depending on a number of known factors and on factors that are not yet fully understood.

What factors increase a woman's risk of breast cancer?

The strongest risk factor for breast cancer is age. A woman's risk of developing this disease increases as she gets older. The risk of breast cancer, however, is not the same for all women in a given age group. Research has shown that women with the following risk factors have an increased chance of developing breast cancer.

- *Genetic alterations (changes)*: Inherited changes in certain genes (including BRCA1, BRCA2, and others) increase the risk of breast cancer. These changes are estimated to account for no more than about 10 percent of all breast cancers. However, women who carry changes in these genes have a much higher risk of breast cancer than women who do not carry these changes.

- *Mammographic breast density*: The glandular (milk-producing) and connective tissue of the breast are mammographically dense—that is, they appear white on a mammogram. In contrast, fatty tissue of the breast is not mammographically dense and appears dark. Women who have a high percentage of breast tissue that appears dense on a mammogram have a higher risk of breast cancer than women of similar age who have little or no dense breast tissue. In general, younger women have denser breasts than older women. As a woman ages, the amount of glandular tissue normally decreases and the amount of fatty tissue increases. Abnormalities, such as tumors, in dense breasts can be more difficult to detect on a mammogram because tumors often also appear white.

- *Family history*: A woman's chance of developing breast cancer increases if her mother, sister, and/or daughter have been diagnosed with the disease, especially if they were diagnosed before age 50. Having a close male blood relative with breast cancer also increases a woman's risk of developing the disease.

- *Personal history of breast cancer*: Women who have had breast cancer are more likely to develop a second breast cancer.

- *Certain breast changes found on biopsy*: Looking at breast tissue under a microscope allows doctors to determine whether a suspicious finding (one detected by a mammogram, for example) represents cancer or another type of breast change. Most breast changes turn out not to be cancer, but some may increase the risk of developing breast cancer. Changes that are associated with an increased risk of breast cancer include atypical hyperplasia (a noncancerous condition in which cells have abnormal features and are increased in number), lobular carcinoma in situ (LCIS) (abnormal cells are found in the lobules of the breast), and ductal carcinoma in situ (DCIS; abnormal cells are found in the lining of breast ducts). Because some cases of DCIS will eventually become cancer, this type of breast change is actively treated. Women with atypical hyperplasia or LCIS are usually monitored carefully and not actively treated. In addition, women who have had two or more breast biopsies for other noncancerous conditions also have an increased risk of developing breast cancer. This increased risk is due to the conditions that led to the biopsies and not to the biopsy procedures themselves.

- *Radiation therapy*: Women who had radiation therapy to the chest (including the breasts) before age 30 have an increased risk of developing breast cancer throughout their lives. This includes women treated for Hodgkin lymphoma. Studies show that the younger a woman was when she received treatment, the higher her risk of developing breast cancer later in life.

- *Alcohol*: Studies indicate that the more alcohol a woman drinks, the greater her risk of breast cancer.

- *Reproductive and menstrual history*: Women who had their first menstrual period before age

12 or who went through menopause after age 55 have an increased risk of developing breast cancer. Women who had their first full-term pregnancy after age 30 or who have never had a full-term pregnancy are also at increased risk of breast cancer.

- *Long-term use of menopausal hormone therapy*: Women who used combined estrogen and progestin menopausal hormone therapy for more than 5 years have an increased chance of developing breast cancer.

- *DES (diethylstilbestrol)*: The drug DES was given to some pregnant women in the United States between 1940 and 1971 to prevent miscarriage. Women who took DES during pregnancy have a slightly increased risk of breast cancer. Women who were exposed to DES in utero—that is, whose mothers took DES while they were pregnant—may have a slightly increased risk of breast cancer after age 40.

- *Body weight*: Studies have found that among postmenopausal women who have not used menopausal hormone therapy, the chance of getting breast cancer is higher in women who are overweight or obese than in women of a healthy weight.

- *Physical activity level:* Women who are physically inactive throughout life may have an increased risk of breast cancer.
- *Race*: In the United States, breast cancer is diagnosed more often in white women than in African American/black, Hispanic/Latina, Asian/Pacific Islander, or American Indian/Alaska Native women.

Chapter 8: Abortion, Miscarriage, and Breast Cancer Risk

Introduction

A woman's hormone levels normally change throughout her life for a variety of reasons, and these hormonal changes can lead to changes in her breasts. Many such hormonal changes occur during pregnancy, changes that may influence a woman's chances of developing breast cancer later in life. As a result, over several decades a considerable amount of research has been and continues to be conducted to determine whether having an induced abortion, or a miscarriage (also known as spontaneous abortion), influences a woman's chances of developing breast cancer later in life.

Current Knowledge

In February 2003, the National Cancer Institute (NCI) convened a workshop of over 100 of the world's leading experts who study pregnancy and breast cancer risk. Workshop participants reviewed existing population-based, clinical, and animal studies on the relationship between pregnancy and breast cancer risk, including studies of induced and spontaneous abortions. They concluded that having an abortion or miscarriage does not increase a woman's subsequent risk of developing breast cancer. NCI regularly reviews and analyzes the scientific literature on many topics, including various risk factors for breast cancer. Considering the body of literature that has been published since 2003, when NCI held this extensive workshop on early reproductive events and cancer, the evidence overall still does not support early termination of pregnancy as a cause of breast cancer.

Background

The relationship between induced and spontaneous abortion and breast cancer risk has been the subject of extensive research beginning in the late 1950s. Until the mid-1990s, the evidence was inconsistent. Findings from some studies suggested there was no increase in risk of breast cancer among women who had had an abortion, while findings from other studies suggested there was an increased risk. Most of these studies, however, were flawed in a number of ways that can lead to unreliable results. Only a small number of women were included in many of these studies, and for most, the data were collected only after breast cancer had been diagnosed, and women's histories of miscarriage and abortion were based on their "self-report" rather than on their medical records. Since then, better-designed studies have been conducted. These newer studies examined large numbers of women, collected data before breast cancer was found, and gathered medical history information from medical records rather than simply from self-reports, thereby generating more reliable findings. The newer studies consistently showed no association between induced and spontaneous abortions and breast cancer risk.

Ongoing Research Supported by the National Cancer Institute

Basic, clinical, and population research will continue to be supported to investigate the relationship and the mechanisms of how hormones in general and during pregnancy influence the development of breast cancer.

Important Information About Breast Cancer Risk Factors

At present, the factors known to increase a woman's chance of developing breast cancer include age (a woman's chances of getting breast cancer increase as she gets older), a family history of breast cancer, an early age at first menstrual period, a late age at menopause, a late age at the time of birth of her first full-term baby, and certain breast conditions. Obesity is also a risk factor for breast cancer in postmenopausal women.

Important Information About Identifying Breast Cancer

NCI recommends that, beginning in their 40s, women receive mammography screening every year or two. Women who have a higher than average risk of breast cancer (for example, women with a family history of breast cancer) should seek expert medical advice about whether they should be screened before age 40, and how frequently they should be screened.

Chapter 9: Reproductive History and Breast Cancer Risk

- The hormonal changes that occur during pregnancy may influence a woman's chance of developing breast cancer later in life.
- Some factors associated with pregnancy may reduce a woman's chance of developing breast cancer later in life.
- Some factors associated with pregnancy may increase a woman's chance of developing breast cancer.
- Induced abortion and miscarriage have not been shown to increase a woman's chance of developing breast cancer.
- Pregnancy may reduce a woman's chance of developing some other cancers, including ovarian and endometrial cancers, later in life.

Is there a relationship between pregnancy and breast cancer risk?

Studies have shown that a woman's risk of developing breast cancer is related to her exposure to hormones that are produced by her ovaries (endogenous estrogen and progesterone). Reproductive factors that increase the duration and/or levels of exposure to ovarian hormones, which stimulate cell growth, have been associated with an increase in breast cancer risk. These factors include early onset of menstruation, late onset of menopause, later age at first pregnancy, and never having given birth.

Pregnancy and breastfeeding both reduce a woman's lifetime number of menstrual cycles, and thus her cumulative exposure to endogenous hormones. In addition, pregnancy and breastfeeding have direct effects on breast cells, causing them to differentiate, or mature, so they can produce milk. Some researchers hypothesize that these differentiated cells are more resistant to becoming transformed into cancer cells than cells that have not undergone differentiation.

Are any pregnancy-related factors associated with a lower risk of breast cancer?

Some pregnancy-related factors have been associated with a reduced risk of developing breast cancer later in life. These factors include the following:

- *Early age at first full-term pregnancy*: Women who have their first full-term pregnancy at an early age have a decreased risk of developing breast cancer later in life. For example, in women who have a first full-term pregnancy before age 20, the risk of developing breast cancer is about half that of women whose first full-term pregnancy occurs after the age of 30. This risk reduction is limited to hormone receptor-positive breast cancer; age at first full-term pregnancy does not appear to affect the risk of hormone receptor-negative breast cancer.

- *Increasing number of births*: The risk of breast cancer declines with the number of children borne. Women who have given birth to five or more children have half the risk of women who have not given birth. Some evidence indicates that the reduced risk associated with an increased number of births may be limited to hormone receptor-positive breast cancer.

- *History of preeclampsia*: Women who have had preeclampsia may have a decreased risk of developing breast cancer. Preeclampsia is a complication of pregnancy in which a woman develops high blood pressure and excess amounts of protein in her urine. Scientists are studying whether certain hormones and proteins associated with preeclampsia may affect breast cancer risk.

- *Longer duration of breastfeeding*: Breastfeeding for an extended period (at least a year) is associated with a decreased risk of both hormone receptor-positive and hormone receptor-negative breast cancer.

Are any pregnancy-related factors associated with an increase in breast cancer risk?

Some factors related to pregnancy may increase the risk of breast cancer. These factors include the following:

- *Older age at birth of first child*: The older a woman is when she has her first full-term pregnancy, the higher her risk of breast cancer. Women who are older than 30 when they give birth to their first child have a higher risk of breast cancer than women who have never given birth.

- *Recent childbirth*: Women who have recently given birth have a short-term increase in risk that declines after about 10 years. The reason for this temporary increase is not known, but some researchers believe that it may be due to the effect of high levels of hormones on microscopic cancers or to the rapid growth of breast cells during pregnancy.

- *Taking diethylstilbestrol (DES) during pregnancy*: Women who took DES during pregnancy have a slightly higher risk of developing breast cancer than women who did not take DES during pregnancy. Daughters of women who took DES during pregnancy may also have a slightly higher risk of developing breast cancer after age 40 than women who were not exposed to DES while in the womb. DES is a synthetic form of estrogen that was used between the early 1940s and 1971 to prevent miscarriages and other pregnancy problems.

Is abortion linked to breast cancer risk?

A few retrospective (case-control) studies reported in the mid-1990s suggested that induced abortion (the deliberate ending of a pregnancy) was associated with an increased risk of breast cancer. However, these studies had important design limitations that could have affected the results. A key limitation was their reliance on self-reporting of medical history information by the study participants, which can introduce bias. Prospective studies, which are more rigorous in design and unaffected by such bias, have consistently shown no association between induced abortion and breast cancer risk. Moreover, in 2009, the Committee on Gynecologic Practice of the American College of Obstetricians and Gynecologists concluded that "more rigorous recent studies demonstrate no causal relationship between induced abortion and a subsequent increase in breast cancer risk". Major findings from these recent studies include the following:

- Women who have had an induced abortion have the same risk of breast cancer as other women.
- Women who have had a spontaneous abortion (miscarriage) have the same risk of breast cancer as other women.
- Cancers other than breast cancer also appear to be unrelated to a history of induced or spontaneous abortion.

Does pregnancy affect the risk of other cancers?

Research has shown the following with regard to pregnancy and the risk of other cancers:

- Women who have had a full-term pregnancy have reduced risks of ovarian and endometrial cancer. Furthermore, the risks of these cancers decline with each additional full-term pregnancy.

- Pregnancy also plays a role in an extremely rare type of tumor called a gestational trophoblastic tumor. In this type of tumor, which starts in the uterus, cancer cells grow in the tissues that are formed following conception.

- There is some evidence that pregnancy-related factors may affect the risk of other cancer types, but these relationships have not been as well studied as those for breast and gynecologic cancers. The associations require further study to clarify the exact relationships.

As in the development of breast cancer, exposures to hormones are thought to explain the role of pregnancy in the development of ovarian, endometrial, and other cancers. Changes in the levels of hormones during pregnancy may contribute to the variation in risk of these tumors after pregnancy.

Chapter 10: Menopausal Hormone Therapy and Cancer

- Much of the evidence about risks and benefits of menopausal hormone therapy (MHT) comes from two randomized clinical trials that were conducted as part of the Women's Health Initiative.

- Although MHT provides short-term benefits, such as relief from hot flashes and vaginal dryness, several health concerns are associated with its use, including increased risk for certain cancers.

- The U.S. Food and Drug Administration currently advises women to use MHT for the shortest time and at the lowest dose possible to control menopausal symptoms.

What is menopausal hormone therapy?

Menopausal hormone therapy (MHT) is a treatment that doctors may recommend to relieve common symptoms of menopause and to address long-term biological changes, such as bone loss, that result from declining levels of the

natural hormones estrogen and progesterone in a woman's body during and after the completion of menopause.
MHT usually involves treatment with estrogen alone, estrogen plus progesterone, or estrogen plus progestin, which is a synthetic hormone with effects similar to those of progesterone. Women who have had a hysterectomy are generally prescribed estrogen alone. Women who have not had this surgery are prescribed estrogen plus progestin, because estrogen alone is associated with an increased risk of endometrial cancer, whereas research has suggested that estrogen plus progestin may not be.

How do the hormones used in MHT differ from the hormones produced by a woman's body?

The hormones used in MHT come from a variety of plants and animals, or they can be made in a laboratory. The chemical structure of these hormones is similar, although usually not identical, to those of hormones produced by women's bodies.

The U.S. Food and Drug Administration (FDA) has approved many hormone products for use in MHT. FDA-approved products have undergone extensive testing and are produced under standardized conditions to ensure that every dose—whether in a pill, a skin patch, or a cream—

contains the proper amount of the appropriate hormones. These FDA-approved products are available only with a doctor's prescription.

Non-FDA-approved hormone products, sometimes referred to as "bio-identical hormones," are widely promoted and sold without a prescription on the Internet. Claims that these products are "safer" or more "natural" than FDA-approved hormonal products are not supported by credible scientific evidence.

Where does evidence about risks and benefits of MHT come from?

The most comprehensive evidence about risks and benefits of MHT comes from two randomized clinical trials that were sponsored by the National Institutes of Health as part of the Women's Health Initiative (WHI):

- The WHI Estrogen-plus-Progestin Study, in which women with a uterus were randomly assigned to receive either a hormone medication containing both estrogen and progestin (Prempro™) or a placebo.
- The WHI Estrogen-Alone Study, in which women without a uterus were randomly assigned to receive either a hormone medication

containing estrogen alone (Premarin™) or a placebo.

More than 27,000 healthy women who were 50 to 79 years of age at the time of enrollment took part in the two trials. Although both trials were stopped early (in 2002 and 2004, respectively) when it was determined that both types of therapy were associated with specific health risks, longer-term follow-up of the participants continues to provide new information about the health effects of MHT.

What are the benefits of MHT?

Research from the WHI Estrogen-plus-Progestin study has shown that women taking combined hormone therapy had the following benefits:

- One-third fewer hip and vertebral fractures than women taking the placebo. In absolute terms, this meant 10 fractures per 10,000 women per year who took hormone therapy compared with 15 fractures per 10,000 women per year who took the placebo.

- One-third lower risk of colorectal cancer than women taking the placebo. In absolute terms, this meant 10 cases of colorectal cancer per 10,000 women per year who took hormone therapy compared with 16 cases of colorectal cancer per 10,000 women per year who took the placebo.

However, a follow-up study found that neither benefit persisted after the study participants stopped taking combined hormone therapy medication.

Women taking estrogen alone experienced the following benefits:

- One-third lower risk for hip and vertebral fractures than women taking the placebo. In absolute terms, this meant 11 hip and 11 vertebral fractures per 10,000 women per year who took estrogen compared with 17 hip and 17 vertebral fractures per 10,000 women per year who took the placebo.

- A 23 percent reduced risk of breast cancer than women taking the placebo. In absolute terms, this meant 26 cases of invasive breast cancer per 10,000 women per year who took estrogen compared with 33 cases of invasive breast cancer per 10,000 women per year who took the placebo.

After 10.7 years of follow-up, however, the risk of hip fractures was slightly higher in the estrogen-alone group, but the risk of breast cancer remained lower than that among women who took the placebo.

What are the health risks of MHT?

Before the WHI studies began, it was known that MHT with estrogen alone increased the risk of endometrial cancer in women with an intact uterus. It was for this reason that, in the WHI trials, women randomly assigned to receive hormone therapy took estrogen plus progestin if they had a uterus and estrogen alone if they didn't have one.

Research from the WHI studies has shown that MHT is associated with the following harms:

- *Urinary incontinence.* Use of estrogen plus progestin increased the risk of urinary incontinence.
- *Dementia.* Use of estrogen plus progestin doubled the risk of developing dementia among postmenopausal women age 65 and older.
- *Stroke, blood clots, and heart attack.* Women who took either combined hormone therapy or estrogen alone had an increased risk of stroke, blood clots, and heart attack. For women in both

groups, however, this risk returned to normal levels after they stopped taking the medication.

- *Breast cancer.* Women who took estrogen plus progestin were more likely to be diagnosed with breast cancer. The breast cancers in these women were larger and more likely to have spread to the lymph nodes by the time they were diagnosed. The number of breast cancers in this group of women increased with the length of time that they took the hormones and decreased after they stopped taking the hormones.

These studies also showed that both combination and estrogen-alone hormone use made mammography less effective for the early detection of breast cancer. Women taking hormones had more repeat mammograms to check on abnormalities found in a screening mammogram and more breast biopsies to determine whether abnormalities detected in mammograms were cancer.

The rate of death from breast cancer among those taking estrogen plus progestin was 2.6 per 10,000 women per year, compared with 1.3 per 10,000 women per year among those taking the placebo. The rate of death from any cause after a diagnosis of breast cancer was 5.3 per 10,000 women per year among women taking combined hormone therapy, compared with 3.4 per 10,000 women per year among those taking the placebo.

- *Lung cancer.* Women who took combined hormone therapy had the same risk of lung cancer as women who took the placebo. However, among those who were diagnosed with lung cancer, women who took estrogen plus progestin were more likely to die of the disease than those who took the placebo. There were no differences in the number of cases or the number of deaths from lung cancer among women who took estrogen alone compared with those among women who took the placebo.

- *Colorectal cancer.* In the initial study report, women taking combined hormone therapy had a lower risk of colorectal cancer than women who took the placebo. However, the colorectal tumors that arose in the combined hormone therapy group were more advanced at detection than those in the placebo group. There was no difference in either the risk of colorectal cancer or the stage of disease at diagnosis between women who took estrogen alone and those who took the placebo.

However, a subsequent analysis of the WHI trials found no strong evidence that either estrogen alone or estrogen plus progestin had any effect on the risk of colorectal cancer, tumor stage at diagnosis, or death from colorectal cancer.

Does hysterectomy affect the cancer risks associated with MHT?

Women who had a hysterectomy and who are prescribed MHT generally take estrogen alone.

In 2004, when the WHI Estrogen-Alone Study was stopped early, women taking estrogen alone had a 23 percent reduced risk of breast cancer compared with those who took the placebo. An analysis conducted after study participants had been followed for an average of 10.7 years found that women who had taken estrogen alone still had a lower risk of breast cancer than women who had taken the placebo.

Do the cancer risks from MHT change over time?

Women who have had a hysterectomy and who use estrogen-alone MHT have a reduced risk of breast cancer that continues for at least 5 years after they stop taking MHT.

Women who take combined hormone therapy have an increased risk of breast cancer that continues after they stop taking the medication. In the WHI study, where women took the combined hormone therapy for an average of 5.6 years, this increased risk persisted after an average follow-up period of 11 years. Breast cancers diagnosed in this group of women were larger and more likely to have spread to the lymph nodes (a sign of more advanced disease). Studies have documented a decline in breast cancer diagnoses in the United States after the sharp reduction in the use of MHT that followed publication of the initial results of the Estrogen-plus-Progestin Study in July 2002. Additional factors, such as a reduction in the use of mammography, may also have contributed to this decline.

Is it safe for women who have had a cancer diagnosis to take MHT?

One of the roles of naturally occurring estrogen is to promote the normal growth of cells in the breast and uterus. For this reason, it is generally believed that MHT may promote further tumor growth in women who have already been diagnosed with breast cancer. However, studies of hormone use to treat menopausal symptoms in breast cancer survivors have produced conflicting results, with some showing an increased risk of breast cancer recurrence and others showing no increased risk of recurrence.

What should women do if they have menopausal symptoms but are concerned about taking MHT?

Although MHT provides short-term benefits such as relief from hot flashes and vaginal dryness, several health concerns, are associated with its use. Women should discuss whether to take MHT and what alternatives may be appropriate for them with their health care provider. The FDA currently advises women to use MHT for the shortest time and at the lowest dose possible to control menopausal symptoms.

Are there alternatives for women who choose not to take MHT?

Women who are concerned about the health effects that occur naturally with the decline in hormone production that occurs during menopause can make changes in their lifestyle and diet to reduce certain risks. For example, eating foods that are rich in calcium and vitamin D or taking dietary supplements containing these nutrients may help to prevent osteoporosis. FDA-approved drugs such as alendronate (Fosamax®), raloxifene (Evista®), and risedronate (Actonel®) have been shown in randomized trials to prevent bone loss.

Medications approved by the FDA for treating depression and seizures may help to relieve menopausal symptoms such as hot flashes (20). Those that have been shown in randomized clinical trials to be effective in treating hot flashes include the following:

- Venlafaxine (Effexor®)
- Desvenlafaxine (Pristiq®)
- Paroxetine (Paxil®)
- Fluoxetine (Prozac®)
- Citalopram (Celexa®)
- Gabapentin (Neurontin®)
- Pregabalin (Lyrica®)

Some women seek relief from menopausal symptoms with over-the-counter complementary and alternative therapies.

Some of these remedies contain estrogen-like compounds derived from sources such as soy products, whole-grain cereals, oilseeds (primarily flaxseed), legumes, or the plant black cohosh. To date, however, randomized clinical trials have not shown that any of these remedies is superior to a placebo in relieving hot flashes. Trials of other herbal remedies, such as evening primrose oil, ginseng, and wild yam, have also not shown that they effectively reduce menopausal symptoms.

Chapter 11: HPV and Cancer

- Some types of sexually transmitted human papillomaviruses (HPVs) can cause genital warts. Other types, called high-risk or oncogenic HPVs, can cause cancer.
- High-risk HPVs cause virtually all cervical cancers. They also cause most anal cancers and some vaginal, vulvar, penile, and oropharyngeal cancers.
- Most infections with high-risk HPVs do not cause cancer. Many HPV infections go away on their own within 1 to 2 years. However, infections that last for many years increase a person's risk of developing cancer.

What are HPVs?

HPVs, also called human papillomaviruses, are a group of more than 150 related viruses. More than 40 of these viruses can be easily spread through direct skin-to-skin contact during vaginal, anal, and oral sex.

HPV infections are the most common sexually transmitted infections in the United States. In fact, more than half of sexually active people are infected with one or more HPV types at some point in their lives. Recent research indicates that, at any point in time, 42.5 percent of women have genital HPV infections, whereas less than 7 percent of adults have oral HPV infections.

Sexually transmitted HPVs fall into two categories:

- Low-risk HPVs, which do not cause cancer but can cause skin warts (technically known as condylomata acuminata) on or around the genitals or anus. For example, HPV types 6 and 11 cause 90 percent of all genital warts.
- High-risk or oncogenic HPVs, which can cause cancer. At least a dozen high-risk HPV types have been identified. Two of these, HPV types 16 and 18, are responsible for the majority of HPV-caused cancers.

What is the association between HPV infection and cancer?

High-risk HPV infection accounts for approximately 5 percent of all cancers worldwide. However, most high-risk HPV infections occur without any symptoms, go away within 1 to 2 years, and do not cause cancer. These transient infections may cause cytologic abnormalities, or abnormal cell changes, that go away on their own.

Some HPV infections, however, can persist for many years. Persistent infections with high-risk HPV types can lead to more serious cytologic abnormalities or lesions that, if untreated, may progress to cancer.

Which cancers are caused by HPVs?

Virtually all cervical cancers are caused by HPV infections, with just two HPV types, 16 and 18, responsible for about 70 percent of all cases. HPV also causes anal cancer, with about 85 percent of all cases caused by HPV-16. HPV types 16 and 18 have also been found to cause close to half of vaginal, vulvar, and penile cancers.

Most recently, HPV infections have been found to cause cancer of the oropharynx, which is the middle part of the throat including the soft palate, the base of the tongue, and the tonsils. In the United States, more than half of the cancers diagnosed in the oropharynx are linked to HPV-16. The incidence of HPV-associated oropharyngeal cancer has increased during the past 20 years, especially among men. It has been estimated that, by 2020, HPV will cause more oropharyngeal cancers than cervical cancers in the United States.

Other factors may increase the risk of developing cancer following a high-risk HPV infection. These other factors include the following:

- Smoking
- Having a weakened immune system
- Having many children (for increased risk of cervical cancer)
- Long-term oral contraceptive use (for increased risk of cervical cancer)
- Poor oral hygiene (for increased risk of oropharyngeal cancer)
- Chronic inflammation

Can HPV infection be prevented?

The most reliable way to prevent infection with either a high-risk or a low-risk HPV is to avoid any skin-to-skin oral, anal, or genital contact with another person. For those who are sexually active, a long-term, mutually monogamous relationship with an uninfected partner is the strategy most likely to prevent HPV infection. However, because of the lack of symptoms it is hard to know whether a partner who has been sexually active in the past is currently infected with HPV.

Research has shown that correct and consistent use of condoms can reduce the transmission of HPVs between sexual partners. Areas not covered by a condom can be infected with the virus, though, so condoms are unlikely to provide complete protection against virus spread.

The Food and Drug Administration (FDA) has approved two HPV vaccines: Gardasil® for the prevention of cervical, anal, vulvar, and vaginal cancer, as well as precancerous lesions in these tissues and genital warts caused by HPV infection; and Cervarix® for the prevention of cervical cancer and precancerous cervical lesions caused by HPV infection. Both vaccines are highly effective in preventing infections with HPV types 16 and 18. Gardasil also prevents infection with HPV types 6 and 11. These vaccines have not been approved for prevention of penile or oropharyngeal cancer.

How are HPV infections detected?

HPV infections can be detected by testing a sample of cells to see if they contain viral DNA or RNA.

The most common test detects DNA from several high-risk HPV types, but it cannot identify the type(s) that are present. Another test is specific for DNA from HPV types 16 and 18, the two types that cause most HPV-associated cancers. A third test can detect DNA from several high-risk HPV types and can indicate whether HPV-16 or HPV-18 is present. A fourth test detects RNA from the most common high-risk HPV types. These tests can detect HPV infections before cell abnormalities are evident.

Theoretically, the HPV DNA and RNA tests could be used to identify HPV infections in cells taken from any part of the body. However, the tests are approved by the FDA for only two indications: for follow-up testing of women who seem to have abnormal Pap test results and for cervical cancer screening in combination with a Pap test among women over age 30.

There are no FDA-approved tests to detect HPV infections in men. There are also no currently recommended screening methods similar to a Pap test for detecting cell changes caused by HPV infection in anal, vulvar, vaginal, penile, or oropharyngeal tissues. However, this is an area of ongoing research.

What are treatment options for HPV-infected individuals?

There is currently no medical treatment for HPV infections. However, the genital warts and precancerous lesions resulting from HPV infections can be treated.

Methods commonly used to treat precancerous cervical lesions include cryosurgery (freezing that destroys tissue), LEEP (loop electrosurgical excision procedure, or the removal of cervical tissue using a hot wire loop), surgical conization (surgery with a scalpel, a laser, or both to remove a cone-shaped piece of tissue from the cervix and cervical canal), and laser vaporization conization (use of a laser to destroy cervical tissue).

Treatments for other types of precancerous lesions caused by HPV (vaginal, vulvar, penile, and anal lesions) and genital warts include topical chemicals or drugs, excisional surgery, cryosurgery, electrosurgery, and laser surgery. HPV-infected individuals who develop cancer generally receive the same treatment as patients whose tumors do not harbor HPV infections, according to the type and stage of their tumors. However, people who are diagnosed with HPV-positive oropharyngeal cancer may be treated differently than people with oropharyngeal cancers that are HPV-negative. Recent research has shown that patients with HPV-positive oropharyngeal tumors have a better prognosis and may do just as well on less intense treatment. An ongoing clinical trial is investigating this question.

How do high-risk HPVs cause cancer?

HPVs infect epithelial cells. These cells, which are organized in layers, cover the inside and outside surfaces of the body, including the skin, the throat, the genital tract, and the anus. Because HPVs are not thought to enter the blood stream, having an HPV infection in one part of the body should not cause an infection in another part of the body.

Once an HPV enters an epithelial cell, the virus begins to make proteins. Two of the proteins made by high-risk HPVs interfere with normal functions in the cell, enabling the cell to grow in an uncontrolled manner and to avoid cell death.

Many times these infected cells are recognized by the immune system and eliminated. Sometimes, however, these infected cells are not destroyed, and a persistent infection results. As the persistently infected cells continue to grow, they may develop mutations that promote even more cell growth, leading to the formation of a high-grade lesion and, ultimately, a tumor.

Researchers believe that it can take between 10 and 20 years from the time of an initial HPV infection until a tumor forms. However, even high-grade lesions do not always lead to cancer. The percentage of high-grade cervical lesions that progress to invasive cervical cancer has been estimated to be 50 percent or less.

Chapter 12: Oral Contraceptives and Cancer Risk

- A number of studies suggest that current use of oral contraceptives (birth control pills) appears to slightly increase the risk of breast cancer, especially among younger women. However, the risk level goes back to normal 10 years or more after discontinuing oral contraceptive use.

- Women who use oral contraceptives have reduced risks of ovarian and endometrial cancer. This protective effect increases with the length of time oral contraceptives are used.

- Oral contraceptive use is associated with an increased risk of cervical cancer; however, this increased risk may be because sexually active women have a higher risk of becoming infected with human papillomavirus, which causes virtually all cervical cancers.

- Women who take oral contraceptives have an increased risk of benign liver tumors, but the relationship between oral contraceptive use and malignant liver tumors is less clear.

What types of oral contraceptives are available in the United States today?

Two types of oral contraceptives (birth control pills) are currently available in the United States. The most commonly prescribed type of oral contraceptive contains man-made versions of the natural female hormones estrogen and progesterone. This type of birth control pill is often called a "combined oral contraceptive." The second type is called the minipill. It contains only progestin, which is the man-made version of progesterone that is used in oral contraceptives.

How could oral contraceptives influence cancer risk?

Naturally occurring estrogen and progesterone have been found to influence the development and growth of some cancers. Because birth control pills contain female hormones, researchers have been interested in determining whether there is any link between these widely used contraceptives and cancer risk.

The results of population studies to examine associations between oral contraceptive use and cancer risk have not always been consistent. Overall, however, the risks of endometrial and ovarian cancer appear to be reduced with the use of oral contraceptives, whereas the risks of breast, cervical, and liver cancer appear to be increased.

How do oral contraceptives affect breast cancer risk?

A woman's risk of developing breast cancer depends on several factors, some of which are related to her natural hormones. Hormonal and reproductive history factors that increase the risk of breast cancer include factors that may allow breast tissue to be exposed to high levels of hormones for longer periods of time, such as the following:

- Beginning menstruation at an early age
- Experiencing menopause at a late age
- Later age at first pregnancy
- Not having children at all

A 1996 analysis of epidemiologic data from more than 50 studies worldwide by the Collaborative Group on Hormonal Factors in Breast Cancer found that women who were current or recent users of birth control pills had a slightly higher risk of developing breast cancer than women who had never used the pill. The risk was highest for women who started using oral contraceptives as teenagers. However, 10 or more years after women stopped using oral contraceptives, their risk of developing breast cancer had returned to the same level as if they had never used birth control pills, regardless of family history of breast cancer, reproductive history, geographic area of residence, ethnic background, differences in study design, dose and type of hormone(s) used, or duration of use. In addition, breast cancers diagnosed in women who had stopped using oral contraceptives for 10 or more years were less advanced than breast cancers diagnosed in women who had never used oral contraceptives.

A recent analysis of data from the Nurses' Health Study, which has been following more than 116,000 female nurses who were 24 to 43 years old when they enrolled in the study in 1989, found that the participants who used oral contraceptives had a slight increase in breast cancer risk. However, nearly all of the increased risk was seen among women who took a specific type of oral contraceptive, a "triphasic" pill, in which the dose of hormones is changed in three stages over the course of a woman's monthly cycle. Because the association with the triphasic formulation was unexpected, more research will be needed to confirm the findings from the Nurses' Health Study.

How do oral contraceptives affect ovarian cancer risks?

Oral contraceptive use has consistently been found to be associated with a reduced risk of ovarian cancer. In a 1992 analysis of 20 studies, researchers found that the longer a woman used oral contraceptives the more her risk of ovarian cancer decreased. The risk decreased by 10 to 12 percent after 1 year of use and by approximately 50 percent after 5 years of use.

Researchers have studied how the amount or type of hormones in oral contraceptives affects ovarian cancer risk. One study, the Cancer and Steroid Hormone (CASH) study, found that the reduction in ovarian cancer risk was the same regardless of the type or amount of estrogen or progestin in the pill. A more recent analysis of data from the CASH study, however, indicated that oral contraceptive formulations with high levels of progestin were associated with a lower risk of ovarian cancer than formulations with low progestin levels. In another study, the Steroid Hormones and Reproductions (SHARE) Study, researchers investigated new, lower-dose progestins that have varying androgenic (testosterone-like) effects. They found no difference in ovarian cancer risk between androgenic and nonandrogenic pills.

Oral contraceptive use by women at increased risk of ovarian cancer due to a genetic mutation in the BRCA1 or

BRCA2 gene has been studied. One study showed a reduction in risk among BRCA1- or BRCA2-mutation carriers who took oral contraceptives, whereas another study showed no effect. A third study, published in 2009, found that women with BRCA1 mutations who took oral contraceptives had about half the risk of ovarian cancer as those who did not.

How do oral contraceptives affect endometrial cancer risk?

Women who use oral contraceptives have been shown to have a reduced risk of endometrial cancer. This protective effect increases with the length of time oral contraceptives are used and continues for many years after a woman stops using oral contraceptives.

How do oral contraceptives affect cervical cancer risk?

Long-term use of oral contraceptives (5 or more years) is associated with an increased risk of cervical cancer. An analysis of 24 epidemiologic studies found that the longer a woman used oral contraceptives, the higher her risk of cervical cancer. However, among women who stopped taking oral contraceptives, the risk tended to decline over time, regardless of how long they had used oral contraceptives before stopping.

In a 2002 report by the International Agency for Research on Cancer, which is part of the World Health Organization, data from eight studies were combined to assess the association between oral contraceptive use and cervical cancer risk among women infected with the human papillomavirus (HPV). Researchers found a nearly threefold increase in risk among women who had used oral contraceptives for 5 to 9 years compared with women who had never used oral contraceptives. Among women who had used oral contraceptives for 10 years or longer, the risk of cervical cancer was four times higher.

Virtually all cervical cancers are caused by persistent infection with high-risk, or oncogenic, types of HPV, and the association of cervical cancer with oral contraceptive use is likely to be indirect. The hormones in oral contraceptives may change the susceptibility of cervical cells to HPV infection, affect their ability to clear the infection, or make it easier for HPV infection to cause changes that progress to cervical cancer. Questions about how oral contraceptives may increase the risk of cervical cancer will be addressed through ongoing research.

How do oral contraceptives affect liver cancer risk?

Oral contraceptive use is associated with an increase in the risk of benign liver tumors, such as hepatocellular adenomas. Benign tumors can form as lumps in different areas of the liver, and they have a high risk of bleeding or rupturing. However, these tumors rarely become malignant. Whether oral contraceptive use increases the risk of malignant liver tumors, also known as hepatocellular carcinomas, is less clear. Some studies have found that women who take oral contraceptives for more than 5 years have an increased risk of hepatocellular carcinoma, but others have not.

Chapter 13: Artificial Sweeteners and Cancer

- Artificial sweeteners are regulated by the U.S. Food and Drug Administration.
- There is no clear evidence that the artificial sweeteners available commercially in the United States are associated with cancer risk in humans.
- Studies have been conducted on the safety of several artificial sweeteners, including saccharin, aspartame, acesulfame potassium, sucralose, neotame, and cyclamate.

What are artificial sweeteners and how are they regulated in the United States?

Artificial sweeteners, also called sugar substitutes, are substances that are used instead of sucrose (table sugar) to sweeten foods and beverages. Because artificial sweeteners are many times sweeter than table sugar, smaller amounts are needed to create the same level of sweetness.

Artificial sweeteners are regulated by the U.S. Food and Drug Administration (FDA). The FDA, like the National Cancer Institute (NCI), is an agency of the Department of

Health and Human Services. The FDA regulates food, drugs, medical devices, cosmetics, biologics, and radiation-emitting products. The Food Additives Amendment to the Food, Drug, and Cosmetic Act, which was passed by Congress in 1958, requires the FDA to approve food additives, including artificial sweeteners, before they can be made available for sale in the United States. However, this legislation does not apply to products that are "generally recognized as safe." Such products do not require FDA approval before being marketed.

Is there an association between artificial sweeteners and cancer?

Questions about artificial sweeteners and cancer arose when early studies showed that cyclamate in combination with saccharin caused bladder cancer in laboratory animals. However, results from subsequent carcinogenicity studies (studies that examine whether a substance can cause cancer) of these sweeteners have not provided clear evidence of an association with cancer in humans. Similarly, studies of other FDA-approved sweeteners have not demonstrated clear evidence of an association with cancer in humans.

What have studies whown about a possible association between specific artificial sweeteners and cancer?

Saccharin

Studies in laboratory rats during the early 1970s linked saccharin with the development of bladder cancer. For this reason, Congress mandated that further studies of saccharin be performed and required that all food containing saccharin bear the following warning label: "Use of this product may be hazardous to your health. This product contains saccharin, which has been determined to cause cancer in laboratory animals."

Subsequent studies in rats showed an increased incidence of urinary bladder cancer at high doses of saccharin, especially in male rats. However, mechanistic studies (studies that examine how a substance works in the body) have shown that these results apply only to rats. Human epidemiology studies (studies of patterns, causes, and control of diseases in groups of people) have shown no consistent evidence that saccharin is associated with bladder cancer incidence.

Because the bladder tumors seen in rats are due to a mechanism not relevant to humans and because there is no clear evidence that saccharin causes cancer in humans, saccharin was delisted in 2000 from the U.S. National Toxicology Program's Report on Carcinogens, where it had been listed since 1981 as a substance reasonably anticipated to be a human carcinogen (a substance known to cause cancer).

Aspartame

Aspartame, distributed under several trade names (e.g., NutraSweet® and Equal®), was approved in 1981 by the FDA after numerous tests showed that it did not cause cancer or other adverse effects in laboratory animals. Questions regarding the safety of aspartame were renewed by a 1996 report suggesting that an increase in the number of people with brain tumors between 1975 and 1992 might be associated with the introduction and use of this sweetener in the United States. However, an analysis of then-current NCI statistics showed that the overall incidence of brain and central nervous system cancers began to rise in 1973, 8 years prior to the approval of aspartame, and continued to rise until 1985. Moreover, increases in overall brain cancer incidence occurred primarily in people age 70 and older, a group that was not exposed to the highest doses of aspartame since its introduction. These data do not establish a clear link between the consumption of aspartame and the development of brain tumors.

In 2005, a laboratory study found more lymphomas and leukemias in rats fed very high doses of aspartame (equivalent to drinking 8 to 2,083 cans of diet soda daily). However, there were some inconsistencies in the findings. For example, the number of cancer cases did not rise with increasing amounts of aspartame as would be expected. Subsequently, NCI examined human data from the NIH-AARP Diet and Health Study of over half a million retirees. Increasing consumption of aspartame-containing beverages was not associated with the development of lymphoma, leukemia, or brain cancer.

Acesulfame potassium, Sucralose, and Neotame

In addition to saccharin and aspartame, three other artificial sweeteners are currently permitted for use in food in the United States:

- Acesulfame potassium (also known as ACK, Sweet One®, and Sunett®) was approved by the FDA in 1988 for use in specific food and beverage categories, and was later approved as a general purpose sweetener (except in meat and poultry) in 2002.

- Sucralose (also known as Splenda®) was approved by the FDA as a tabletop sweetener in 1998, followed by approval as a general purpose sweetener in 1999.
- Neotame, which is similar to aspartame, was approved by the FDA as a general purpose sweetener (except in meat and poultry) in 2002.

Before approving these sweeteners, the FDA reviewed more than 100 safety studies that were conducted on each sweetener, including studies to assess cancer risk. The results of these studies showed no evidence that these sweeteners cause cancer or pose any other threat to human health.

Cyclamate

Because the findings in rats suggested that cyclamate might increase the risk of bladder cancer in humans, the FDA banned the use of cyclamate in 1969. After reexamination of cyclamate's carcinogenicity and the evaluation of additional data, scientists concluded that cyclamate was not a carcinogen or a co-carcinogen (a substance that enhances the effect of a cancer-causing substance). A food additive petition was filed with the FDA for the reapproval of cyclamate, but this petition is currently being held in abeyance (not actively being considered). The FDA's concerns about cyclamate are not cancer related.

Chapter 14: Chemicals in Meat Cooked at High Temperatures and Cancer Risk

- Heterocyclic amines (HCAs) and polycyclic aromatic hydrocarbons (PAHs) are chemicals formed when muscle meat, including beef, pork, fish, and poultry, is cooked using high-temperature methods, such as pan frying or grilling directly over an open flame.

- The formation of HCAs and PAHs is influenced by the type of meat, the cooking time, the cooking temperature, and the cooking method.

- Exposure to high levels of HCAs and PAHs can cause cancer in animals; however, whether such exposure causes cancer in humans is unclear.

- Currently, no Federal guidelines address consumption levels of HCAs and PAHs formed in meat.

- HCA and PAH formation can be reduced by avoiding direct exposure of meat to an open flame or a hot metal surface, reducing the cooking time, and using a microwave oven to partially cook meat before exposing it to high temperatures.

- Ongoing studies are investigating the associations between meat intake, meat cooking methods, and cancer risk.

What are heterocyclic amines and polycyclic aromatic hydrocarbons, and how are they formed in cooked meats?

Heterocyclic amines (HCAs) and polycyclic aromatic hydrocarbons (PAHs) are chemicals formed when muscle meat, including beef, pork, fish, or poultry, is cooked using high-temperature methods, such as pan frying or grilling directly over an open flame. In laboratory experiments, HCAs and PAHs have been found to be mutagenic—that is, they cause changes in DNA that may increase the risk of cancer.

HCAs are formed when amino acids (the building blocks of proteins), sugars, and creatine (a substance found in muscle) react at high temperatures. PAHs are formed when fat and juices from meat grilled directly over an open fire drip onto the fire, causing flames. These flames contain PAHs that then adhere to the surface of the meat. PAHs can also be formed during other food preparation processes, such as smoking of meats.

HCAs are not found in significant amounts in foods other than meat cooked at high temperatures. PAHs can be found in other charred foods, as well as in cigarette smoke and car exhaust fumes.

What factors influence the formation of HCA and PAH in cooked meats?

The formation of HCAs and PAHs varies by meat type, cooking method, and "doneness" level (rare, medium, or well done). Whatever the type of meat, however, meats cooked at high temperatures, especially above 300°F (as in grilling or pan frying), or that are cooked for a long time tend to form more HCAs. For example, well done, grilled, or barbecued chicken and steak all have high concentrations of HCAs. Cooking methods that expose meat to smoke or charring contribute to PAH formation. HCAs and PAHs become capable of damaging DNA only after they are metabolized by specific enzymes in the body, a process called "bioactivation." Studies have found that the activity of these enzymes, which can differ among people, may be relevant to cancer risks associated with exposure to these compounds.

What evidence is there that HCAs and PAHs in cooked meats may increase cancer risk?

Studies have shown that exposure to HCAs and PAHs can cause cancer in animal models. In many experiments, rodents fed a diet supplemented with HCAs developed tumors of the breast, colon, liver, skin, lung, prostate, and other organs. Rodents fed PAHs also developed cancers, including leukemia and tumors of the gastrointestinal tract and lungs. However, the doses of HCAs and PAHs used in these studies were very high—equivalent to thousands of times the doses that a person would consume in a normal diet.

Population studies have not established a definitive link between HCA and PAH exposure from cooked meats and cancer in humans. One difficulty with conducting such studies is that it can be difficult to determine the exact level of HCA and/or PAH exposure a person gets from cooked meats. Although dietary questionnaires can provide good estimates, they may not capture all the detail about cooking techniques that is necessary to determine HCA and PAH exposure levels. In addition, individual variation in the activity of enzymes that metabolize HCAs and PAHs may result in exposure differences, even among people who ingest (take in) the same amount of these compounds. Also, people may have been exposed to PAHs from other environmental sources, such as pollution and tobacco smoke.

Nevertheless, numerous epidemiologic studies have used detailed questionnaires to examine participants' meat consumption and meat cooking methods to estimate HCA and PAH exposures. Researchers found that high consumption of well-done, fried, or barbecued meats was associated with increased risks of colorectal, pancreatic, and prostate cancer.

Do guidelines exist for the consumption of food containing HCAs and PAHs?

Currently, no Federal guidelines address the consumption of foods containing HCAs and PAHs. The World Cancer Research Fund/American Institute for Cancer Research issued a report in 2007 with dietary guidelines that recommended limiting the consumption of red and processed (including smoked) meats; however, no recommendations were provided for HCA and PAH levels in meat.

Are there ways to reduce HCA and PAH formation in cooked meats?

Even though no specific guidelines for HCA/PAH consumption exist, concerned individuals can reduce their exposure by using several cooking methods:

- Avoiding direct exposure of meat to an open flame or a hot metal surface and avoiding prolonged cooking times (especially at high temperatures) can help reduce HCA and PAH formation.

- Using a microwave oven to cook meat prior to exposure to high temperatures can also substantially reduce HCA formation by reducing the time that meat must be in contact with high heat to finish cooking.

- Continuously turning meat over on a high heat source can substantially reduce HCA formation compared with just leaving the meat on the heat source without flipping it often.

- Removing charred portions of meat and refraining from using gravy made from meat drippings can also reduce HCA and PAH exposure.

What research is being conducted on the relationship between the consumption of HCAs and PAHs and cancer risk in humans?

Researchers in the United States are currently investigating the association between meat intake, meat cooking methods, and cancer risk. Ongoing studies include the NIH-AARP Diet and Health Study, the American Cancer Society's Cancer Prevention Study II, the Multiethnic Cohort, and studies from Harvard University. Similar research in a European population is being conducted in the European Prospective Investigation into Cancer and Nutrition (EPIC) study.

Chapter 15: Asbestos Exposure and Cancer Risk

- Asbestos is the name given to a group of minerals that occur naturally in the environment as bundles of fibers.

- Exposure to asbestos may increase the risk of asbestosis, other nonmalignant lung and pleural disorders, lung cancer, mesothelioma, and other cancers.

- Smokers who are also exposed to asbestos have a greatly increased risk of lung cancer.

- Individuals who have been exposed (or suspect they have been exposed) to asbestos on the job, through the environment, or at home through a family contact should inform their physician and report any symptoms.

- Government agencies can provide additional information on asbestos exposure.

What is asbestos?

Asbestos is the name given to a group of minerals that occur naturally in the environment as bundles of fibers that can be separated into thin, durable threads. These fibers are resistant to heat, fire, and chemicals and do not conduct electricity. For these reasons, asbestos has been used widely in many industries.

Chemically, asbestos minerals are silicate compounds, meaning they contain atoms of silicon and oxygen in their molecular structure.

Asbestos minerals are divided into two major groups: Serpentine asbestos and amphibole asbestos. Serpentine asbestos includes the mineral chrysotile, which has long, curly fibers that can be woven. Chrysotile asbestos is the form that has been used most widely in commercial applications. Amphibole asbestos includes the minerals actinolite, tremolite, anthophyllite, crocidolite, and amosite. Amphibole asbestos has straight, needle-like fibers that are more brittle than those of serpentine asbestos and are more limited in their ability to be fabricated.

How is asbestos used?

Asbestos has been mined and used commercially in North America since the late 1800s. Its use increased greatly during World War II. Since then, asbestos has been used in many industries. For example, the building and construction industries have used it for strengthening cement and plastics as well as for insulation, roofing, fireproofing, and sound absorption. The shipbuilding industry has used asbestos to insulate boilers, steam pipes, and hot water pipes. The automotive industry uses asbestos in vehicle brake shoes and clutch pads. Asbestos has also been used in ceiling and floor tiles; paints, coatings, and adhesives; and plastics. In addition, asbestos has been found in vermiculite-containing garden products and some talc-containing crayons.

In the late 1970s, the U.S. Consumer Product Safety Commission (CPSC) banned the use of asbestos in wallboard patching compounds and gas fireplaces because the asbestos fibers in these products could be released into the environment during use. In addition, manufacturers of electric hairdryers voluntarily stopped using asbestos in their products in 1979. In 1989, the U.S. Environmental Protection Agency (EPA) banned all new uses of asbestos; however, uses developed before 1989 are still allowed. The EPA also established regulations that require school systems to inspect buildings for the presence of damaged asbestos and to eliminate or reduce asbestos exposure to occupants by removing the asbestos or encasing it.

In June 2000, the CPSC concluded that the risk of children's exposure to asbestos fibers in crayons was extremely low. However, U.S. manufacturers of these crayons agreed to eliminate talc from their products.

In August 2000, the EPA conducted a series of tests to evaluate the risk for consumers of adverse health effects associated with exposure to asbestos-contaminated vermiculite. The EPA concluded that exposure to asbestos from some vermiculite products poses only a minimal health risk. The EPA recommended that consumers reduce the low risk associated with the occasional use of vermiculite during gardening activities by limiting the amount of dust produced during vermiculite use. Specifically, the EPA suggested that consumers use vermiculite outdoors or in a well-ventilated area; keep vermiculite damp while using it; avoid bringing dust from vermiculite into the home on clothing; and use premixed potting soil, which is less likely to generate dust.

The regulations described above and other actions, coupled with widespread public concern about the health hazards of asbestos, have resulted in a significant annual decline in the U.S. use of asbestos. Domestic consumption of asbestos amounted to about 803,000 metric tons in 1973, but it had dropped to about 2,400 metric tons by 2005.

What are the health hazards of exposure to asbestos?

People may be exposed to asbestos in their workplace, their communities, or their homes. If products containing asbestos are disturbed, tiny asbestos fibers are released into the air. When asbestos fibers are breathed in, they may get trapped in the lungs and remain there for a long time. Over time, these fibers can accumulate and cause scarring and inflammation, which can affect breathing and lead to serious health problems.

Asbestos has been classified as a known human carcinogen (a substance that causes cancer) by the U.S. Department of Health and Human Services, the EPA, and the International Agency for Research on Cancer. Studies have shown that exposure to asbestos may increase the risk of lung cancer and mesothelioma (a relatively rare cancer of the thin membranes that line the chest and abdomen). Although rare, mesothelioma is the most common form of cancer associated with asbestos exposure. In addition to lung cancer and mesothelioma, some studies have suggested an association between asbestos exposure and gastrointestinal and colorectal cancers, as well as an elevated risk for cancers of the throat, kidney, esophagus, and gallbladder. However, the evidence is inconclusive.

Asbestos exposure may also increase the risk of asbestosis (an inflammatory condition affecting the lungs that can cause shortness of breath, coughing, and permanent lung damage) and other nonmalignant lung and pleural disorders, including pleural plaques (changes in the membranes surrounding the lung), pleural thickening, and benign pleural effusions (abnormal collections of fluid between the thin layers of tissue lining the lungs and the wall of the chest cavity). Although pleural plaques are not precursors to lung cancer, evidence suggests that people with pleural disease caused by exposure to asbestos may be at increased risk for lung cancer.

Who is at risk for an asbestos-related disease?

Everyone is exposed to asbestos at some time during their life. Low levels of asbestos are present in the air, water, and soil. However, most people do not become ill from their exposure. People who become ill from asbestos are usually those who are exposed to it on a regular basis, most often in a job where they work directly with the material or through substantial environmental contact.

Since the early 1940s, millions of American workers have been exposed to asbestos. Health hazards from asbestos fibers have been recognized in workers exposed in the shipbuilding trades, asbestos mining and milling, manufacturing of asbestos textiles and other asbestos products, insulation work in the construction and building trades, and a variety of other trades. Demolition workers, drywall removers, asbestos removal workers, firefighters, and automobile workers also may be exposed to asbestos fibers. Studies evaluating the cancer risk experienced by automobile mechanics exposed to asbestos through brake repair are limited, but the overall evidence suggests there is no safe level of asbestos exposure. As a result of Government regulations and improved work practices, today's workers (those without previous exposure) are likely to face smaller risks than did those exposed in the past.

Individuals involved in the rescue, recovery, and cleanup at the site of the September 11, 2001, attacks on the World Trade Center (WTC) in New York City are another group at risk of developing an asbestos-related disease. Because asbestos was used in the construction of the North Tower of the WTC, when the building was attacked, hundreds of tons of asbestos were released into the atmosphere. Those at greatest risk include firefighters, police officers, paramedics, construction workers, and volunteers who worked in the rubble at Ground Zero. Others at risk include residents in close proximity to the WTC towers and those who attended schools nearby. These individuals will need to be followed to determine the long-term health consequences of their exposure.

One study found that nearly 70 percent of WTC rescue and recovery workers suffered new or worsened respiratory symptoms while performing work at the WTC site. The study describes the results of the WTC Worker and Volunteer Medical Screening Program, which was established to identify and characterize possible WTC-related health effects in responders. The study found that about 28 percent of those tested had abnormal lung function tests, and 61 percent of those without previous health problems developed respiratory symptoms. However, it is important to note that these symptoms may be related to exposure to debris components other than asbestos.

Although it is clear that the health risks from asbestos exposure increase with heavier exposure and longer exposure time, investigators have found asbestos-related diseases in individuals with only brief exposures. Generally, those who develop asbestos-related diseases show no signs of illness for a long time after their first exposure. It can take from 10 to 40 years or more for symptoms of an asbestos-related condition to appear. There is some evidence that family members of workers heavily exposed to asbestos face an increased risk of developing mesothelioma. This risk is thought to result from exposure to asbestos fibers brought into the home on the shoes, clothing, skin, and hair of workers. To decrease these exposures, Federal law regulates workplace practices to limit the possibility of asbestos being brought home in this way. Some employees may be required to shower and change their clothes before they leave work, store their street clothes in a separate area of the workplace, or wash their work clothes at home separately from other clothes. Cases of mesothelioma have also been seen in individuals without occupational asbestos exposure who live close to asbestos mines.

What factors affect the risk of developing an asbestos-related disease?

Several factors can help to determine how asbestos exposure affects an individual, including:

- Dose (how much asbestos an individual was exposed to).
- Duration (how long an individual was exposed).

- Size, shape, and chemical makeup of the asbestos fibers.
- Source of the exposure.
- Individual risk factors, such as smoking and pre-existing lung disease.

Although all forms of asbestos are considered hazardous, different types of asbestos fibers may be associated with different health risks. For example, the results of several studies suggest that amphibole forms of asbestos may be more harmful than chrysotile, particularly for mesothelioma risk, because they tend to stay in the lungs for a longer period of time.

How does smoking affect risk?

Many studies have shown that the combination of smoking and asbestos exposure is particularly hazardous. Smokers who are also exposed to asbestos have a risk of developing lung cancer that is greater than the individual risks from asbestos and smoking added together. There is evidence that quitting smoking will reduce the risk of lung cancer among asbestos-exposed workers. Smoking combined with asbestos exposure does not appear to increase the risk of mesothelioma. However, people who were exposed to asbestos on the job at any time during their life or who suspect they may have been exposed should not smoke.

How are asbestos-related diseases detected?

Individuals who have been exposed (or suspect they have been exposed) to asbestos fibers on the job, through the environment, or at home via a family contact should inform their doctor about their exposure history and whether or not they experience any symptoms. The symptoms of asbestos-related diseases may not become apparent for many decades after the exposure. It is particularly important to check with a doctor if any of the following symptoms develop:

- Shortness of breath, wheezing, or hoarseness.
- A persistent cough that gets worse over time.
- Blood in the sputum (fluid) coughed up from the lungs.
- Pain or tightening in the chest.
- Difficulty swallowing.
- Swelling of the neck or face.
- Loss of appetite.
- Weight loss.
- Fatigue or anemia.

A thorough physical examination, including a chest x-ray and lung function tests, may be recommended. The chest x-ray is currently the most common tool used to detect asbestos-related diseases. However, it is important to note that chest x-rays cannot detect asbestos fibers in the lungs, but they can help identify any early signs of lung disease resulting from asbestos exposure.

Studies have shown that computed tomography (CT) (a series of detailed pictures of areas inside the body taken from different angles; the pictures are created by a computer linked to an x-ray machine) may be more effective than conventional chest x-rays at detecting asbestos-related lung abnormalities in individuals who have been exposed to asbestos.

A lung biopsy, which detects microscopic asbestos fibers in pieces of lung tissue removed by surgery, is the most reliable test to confirm the presence of asbestos-related abnormalities. A bronchoscopy is a less invasive test than a biopsy and detects asbestos fibers in material that is rinsed out of the lungs. It is important to note that these tests cannot determine how much asbestos an individual may have been exposed to or whether disease will develop. Asbestos fibers can also be detected in urine, mucus, or feces, but these tests are not reliable for determining how much asbestos may be in an individual's lungs.

How can workers protect themselves from asbestos exposure?

The Occupational Safety and Health Administration (OSHA) is a component of the U.S. Department of Labor (DOL) and is the Federal agency responsible for health and safety regulations in maritime, construction, manufacturing, and service workplaces. OSHA established regulations dealing with asbestos exposure on the job, specifically in construction work, shipyards, and general industry, that employers are required to follow. In addition, the Mine Safety and Health Administration (MSHA), another component of the DOL, enforces regulations related to mine safety. Workers should use all protective equipment provided by their employers and follow recommended workplace practices and safety procedures. For example, National Institute for Occupational Safety and Health (NIOSH)-approved respirators that fit properly should be worn by workers when required.

Workers who are concerned about asbestos exposure in the workplace should discuss the situation with other employees, their employee health and safety representative, and their employers. If necessary, OSHA can provide more information or make an inspection.

Chapter 16: Cell Phones and Cancer Risk

- Cell phones emit radiofrequency energy, a form of non-ionizing electromagnetic radiation, which can be absorbed by tissues closest to where the phone is held.

- The amount of radiofrequency energy a cell phone user is exposed to depends on the technology of the phone, the distance between the phone's antenna and the user, the extent and type of use, and the user's distance from cell phone towers.

- Studies thus far have not shown a consistent link between cell phone use and cancers of the brain, nerves, or other tissues of the head or neck. More research is needed because cell phone technology and how people use cell phones have been changing rapidly.

Why is there concern that cell phones may cause cancer or other health problems?

There are three main reasons why people are concerned that cell phones (also known as "wireless" or "mobile" telephones) might have the potential to cause certain types of cancer or other health problems:

- Cell phones emit radiofrequency energy (radio waves), a form of non-ionizing radiation. Tissues nearest to where the phone is held can absorb this energy.

- The number of cell phone users has increased rapidly. As of 2010, there were more than 303 million subscribers to cell phone service in the United States, according to the Cellular Telecommunications and Internet Association. This is a nearly threefold increase from the 110 million users in 2000. Globally, the number of cell phone subscriptions is estimated by the International Telecommunications Union to be 5 billion.

- Over time, the number of cell phone calls per day, the length of each call, and the amount of time people use cell phones have increased. Cell phone technology has also undergone substantial changes.

What is radiofrequency energy and how does it affect the body?

Radiofrequency energy is a form of electromagnetic radiation. Electromagnetic radiation can be categorized into two types: ionizing (e.g., x-rays, radon, and cosmic rays) and non-ionizing (e.g., radiofrequency and extremely low-frequency or power frequency).

Exposure to ionizing radiation, such as from radiation therapy, is known to increase the risk of cancer. However, although many studies have examined the potential health effects of non-ionizing radiation from radar, microwave ovens, and other sources, there is currently no consistent evidence that non-ionizing radiation increases cancer risk.

The only known biological effect of radiofrequency energy is heating. The ability of microwave ovens to heat food is one example of this effect of radiofrequency energy. Radiofrequency exposure from cell phone use does cause heating; however, it is not sufficient to measurably increase body temperature.

A recent study showed that when people used a cell phone for 50 minutes, brain tissues on the same side of the head as the phone's antenna metabolized more glucose than did tissues on the opposite side of the brain. The researchers noted that the results are preliminary, and possible health outcomes from this increase in glucose metabolism are still unknown.

What has research shown about the possible cancer-causing effects of radiofrequency energy?

Although there have been some concerns that radiofrequency energy from cell phones held closely to the head may affect the brain and other tissues, to date there is no evidence from studies of cells, animals, or humans that radiofrequency energy can cause cancer.

It is generally accepted that damage to DNA is necessary for cancer to develop. However, radiofrequency energy, unlike ionizing radiation, does not cause DNA damage in cells, and it has not been found to cause cancer in animals or to enhance the cancer-causing effects of known chemical carcinogens in animals.

Researchers have carried out several types of epidemiologic studies to investigate the possibility of a relationship between cell phone use and the risk of malignant (cancerous) brain tumors, such as gliomas, as well as benign (noncancerous) tumors, such as acoustic neuromas (tumors in the cells of the nerve responsible for hearing), most meningiomas (tumors in the meninges, membranes that cover and protect the brain and spinal cord), and parotid gland tumors (tumors in the salivary glands).

In one type of study, called a case-control study, cell phone use is compared between people with these types of tumors and people without them. In another type of study, called a cohort study, a large group of people is followed over time and the rate of these tumors in people who did and didn't use cell phones is compared. Cancer incidence data can also be analyzed over time to see if the rates of cancer changed in large populations during the time that cell phone use increased dramatically. The results of these studies have generally not provided clear evidence of a relationship between cell phone use and cancer, but there have been some statistically significant findings in certain subgroups of people.

Findings from specific research studies are summarized below:

- The Interphone Study, conducted by a consortium of researchers from 13 countries, is the largest health-related case-control study of use of cell phones and head and neck tumors. Most published analyses from this study have shown no statistically significant increases in brain or central nervous system cancers related to higher amounts of cell phone use. One recent analysis showed a statistically significant, albeit modest, increase in the risk of glioma among the small proportion of study participants who spent the most total time on cell phone calls. However, the researchers considered this finding inconclusive because they felt that the amount of use reported by some respondents was unlikely and because the participants who reported lower levels of use appeared to have a reduced risk of brain cancer. Another recent study from the group found no relationship between brain tumor locations and regions of the brain that were exposed to the highest level of radiofrequency energy from cell phones.

- A cohort study in Denmark linked billing information from more than 358,000 cell phone subscribers with brain tumor incidence data from the Danish Cancer Registry. The analyses found no association between cell phone use and the incidence of glioma, meningioma, or acoustic neuroma, even among people who had been cell phone subscribers for 13 or more years.

- Early case-control studies in the United States, Europe, and Japan were unable to demonstrate a relationship between cell phone use and glioma or meningioma.

- Some case-control studies in Sweden found statistically significant trends of increasing brain cancer risk for the total amount of cell phone use and the years of use among people who began using cell phones before age 20. However, another large, case-control study in Sweden did not find an increased risk of brain cancer among people between the ages of 20 and 69. In addition, the international CEFALO study, which compared children who were diagnosed with brain cancer between ages 7 and 19 with similar children who were not, found no relationship between their cell phone use and risk for brain cancer.

- NCI's Surveillance, Epidemiology, and End Results (SEER) Program, which tracks cancer incidence in the United States over time, found no increase in the incidence of brain or other central nervous system cancers between 1987 and 2007, despite the dramatic increase in cell phone use in this country during that time. Similarly, incidence data from Denmark,

Finland, Norway, and Sweden for the period 1974–2008 revealed no increase in age-adjusted incidence of brain tumors. A 2012 study by NCI researchers, which compared observed glioma incidence rates in SEER with projected rates based on risks observed in the Interphone study, found that the projected rates were consistent with observed U.S. rates. The researchers also compared the SEER rates with projected rates based on a Swedish study published in 2011. They determined that the projected rates were at least 40 percent higher than, and incompatible with, the actual U.S. rates.

- Studies of workers exposed to radiofrequency energy have shown no evidence of increased risk of brain tumors among U.S. Navy electronics technicians, aviation technicians, or fire control technicians, those working in an electromagnetic pulse test program, plastic-ware workers, cellular phone manufacturing workers, or Navy personnel with a high probability of exposure to radar.

Why are the findings from different studies of cell phone use and cancer risk inconsistent?

A limited number of studies have shown some evidence of statistical association of cell phone use and brain tumor risks, but most studies have found no association. Reasons for these discrepancies include the following:

- *Recall bias*, which may happen when a study collects data about prior habits and exposures using questionnaires administered after disease has been diagnosed in some of the study participants. It is possible that study participants who have brain tumors may remember their cell phone use differently than individuals without brain tumors. Many epidemiologic studies of cell phone use and brain cancer risk lack verifiable data about the total amount of cell phone use over time. In addition, people who develop a brain tumor may have a tendency to recall using their cell phone mostly on the same side of their head where the tumor was found, regardless of whether they actually used their phone on that side of their head a lot or only a little.

- *Inaccurate reporting*, which may happen when people say that something has happened more or less often than it actually did. People may not remember how much they used cell phones in a given time period.

- *Morbidity and mortality* among study participants who have brain cancer. Gliomas are particularly difficult to study, for example, because of their high death rate and the short survival of people who develop these tumors. Patients who survive initial treatment are often impaired, which may affect their responses to questions. Furthermore, for people who have died, next-of-kin are often less familiar with the cell phone use patterns of their deceased family member and may not accurately describe their patterns of use to an interviewer.

- *Participation bias*, which can happen when people who are diagnosed with brain tumors are more likely than healthy people (known as controls) to enroll in a research study. Also, controls who did not or rarely used cell phones were less likely to participate in the Interphone study than controls who used cell phones regularly. For example, the Interphone study reported participation rates of 78 percent for meningioma patients (range 56–92 percent for the individual studies), 64 percent for the glioma patients (range 36–92 percent), and 53 percent for control subjects (range 42–74 percent) (9). One series of Swedish studies reported participation rates of 85 percent in people with brain cancer and 84 percent in control subjects.

- *Changing technology and methods of use.* Older studies evaluated radiofrequency energy exposure from analog cell phones. However, most cell phones today use digital technology, which operates at a different frequency and a lower power level than analog phones. Digital cell phones have been in use for more than a decade in the United States, and cellular technology continues to change. Texting, for example, has become a popular way of using a cell phone to communicate that does not require bringing the phone close to the head. Furthermore, the use of hands-free technology, such as wired and wireless headsets, is increasing and may decrease radiofrequency energy exposure to the head and brain.

What do expert organizations conclude?

The International Agency for Research on Cancer (IARC), a component of the World Health Organization, has recently classified radiofrequency fields as "possibly carcinogenic to humans," based on limited evidence from human studies, limited evidence from studies of radiofrequency energy and cancer in rodents, and weak mechanistic evidence (from studies of genotoxicity, effects on immune system function, gene and protein expression, cell signaling, oxidative stress, and apoptosis, along with studies of the possible effects of radiofrequency energy on the blood-brain barrier).

The American Cancer Society (ACS) states that the IARC classification means that there could be some risk associated with cancer, but the evidence is not strong enough to be considered causal and needs to be investigated further. Individuals who are concerned about radiofrequency exposure can limit their exposure, including using an ear piece and limiting cell phone use, particularly among children.

The National Institute of Environmental Health Sciences (NIEHS) states that the weight of the current scientific evidence has not conclusively linked cell phone use with any adverse health problems, but more research is needed. The U.S. Food and Drug Administration (FDA), which is responsible for regulating the safety of machines and devices that emit radiation (including cell phones), notes that studies reporting biological changes associated with radiofrequency energy have failed to be replicated and that the majority of human epidemiologic studies have failed to show a relationship between exposure to radiofrequency energy from cell phones and health problems. The U.S. Centers for Disease Control and Prevention (CDC) states that, although some studies have raised concerns about the possible risks of cell phone use, scientific research as a whole does not support a statistically significant association between cell phone use and health effects. The Federal Communications Commission (FCC) concludes that there is no scientific evidence that proves that wireless phone use can lead to cancer or to other health problems, including headaches, dizziness, or memory loss.

Do children have a higher risk of developing cancer due to cell phone use than adults?

In theory, children have the potential to be at greater risk than adults for developing brain cancer from cell phones. Their nervous systems are still developing and therefore more vulnerable to factors that may cause cancer. Their heads are smaller than those of adults and therefore have a greater proportional exposure to the field of radiofrequency radiation that is emitted by cell phones. And children have the potential of accumulating more years of cell phone exposure than adults do.

So far, the data from clinical studies in children do not support this theory. The first published analysis came from a large case-control study called CEFALO, which was conducted in Denmark, Sweden, Norway, and Switzerland. The study included children who were diagnosed with brain tumors between 2004 and 2008, when their ages ranged from 7 to 19. Researchers did not find an association between cell phone use and brain tumor risk in this group of children. However, they noted that their results did not rule out the possibility of a slight increase in brain cancer risk among children who use cell phones, and that data gathered through prospective studies and objective measurements, rather than participant surveys and recollections, will be key in clarifying whether there is an increased risk.

Researchers from the Centre for Research in Environmental Epidemiology in Spain are conducting another international study—Mobi-Kids —to evaluate the risk associated with new communications technologies (including cell phones) and other environmental factors in young people ages 10 to 24.

What can cell phone users do to reduce their exposure to radiofrequency energy?

The FDA and FCC have suggested some steps that concerned cell phone users can take to reduce their exposure to radiofrequency energy:

- Reserve the use of cell phones for shorter conversations or for times when a landline phone is not available.
- Use a hands-free device, which places more distance between the phone and the head of the user.

Hands-free kits reduce the amount of radiofrequency energy exposure to the head because the antenna, which is the source of energy, is not placed against the head.

Chapter 17: Common Moles, Dysplastic Nevi, and Risk of Melanoma

- A common mole (nevus) is a small growth on the skin that is usually pink, tan, or brown and has a distinct edge. People who have more than 50 common moles have a greater chance than others of developing a dangerous type of skin cancer known as melanoma. Most common moles do not turn into melanoma.

- A dysplastic nevus is an unusual mole that is often large and flat and does not have a symmetric round or oval shape. The edge is often indistinct. It may have a mixture of pink, tan, or brown shades. People who have many dysplastic nevi have a greater chance than others of developing melanoma, but most dysplastic nevi do not turn into melanoma.

- If the color, size, shape, or height of a mole changes or if it starts to itch, bleed, or ooze, people should tell their doctor. People should also tell their doctor if they see a new mole that doesn't look like their other moles.

- The only way to diagnose melanoma is to remove tissue and check it for cancer cells.

What is a common mole?

A common mole is a growth on the skin that develops when pigment cells (melanocytes) grow in clusters. Most adults have between 10 and 40 common moles. These growths are usually found above the waist on areas exposed to the sun. They are seldom found on the scalp, breast, or buttocks.

Although common moles may be present at birth, they usually appear later in childhood. Most people continue to develop new moles until about age 40. In older people, common moles tend to fade away.

Another name for a mole is a nevus. The plural is nevi.

What does a common mole look like?

A common mole is usually smaller than about 5 millimeters wide (about 1/4 inch, the width of a pencil eraser). It is round or oval, has a smooth surface with a distinct edge, and is often dome-shaped. A common mole usually has an even color of pink, tan, or brown. People who have dark skin or hair tend to have darker moles than people with fair skin or blonde hair.

Can a common mole turn into melanoma?

Yes, but a common mole rarely turns into melanoma, which is the most serious type of skin cancer.

Although common moles are not cancerous, people who have more than 50 common moles have an increased chance of developing melanoma.

People should tell their doctor if they notice any of the following changes in a common mole:

- The color changes
- The mole gets unevenly smaller or bigger (unlike normal moles in children, which get evenly bigger)
- The mole changes in shape, texture, or height
- The skin on the surface becomes dry or scaly
- The mole becomes hard or feels lumpy
- It starts to itch
- It bleeds or oozes

What is a dysplastic nevus?

A dysplastic nevus is a type of mole that looks different from a common mole. (Some doctors use the term "atypical mole" to refer to a dysplastic nevus.) A dysplastic nevus may be bigger than a common mole, and its color, surface, and border may be different. It is usually more than 5 millimeters wide. A dysplastic nevus can have a mixture of several colors, from pink to dark brown. Usually, it is flat with a smooth, slightly scaly, or pebbly surface, and it has an irregular edge that may fade into the surrounding skin. A dysplastic nevus may occur anywhere on the body, but it is usually seen in areas exposed to the sun, such as on the back. A dysplastic nevus may also appear in areas not exposed to the sun, such as the scalp, breasts, and areas below the waist. Some people have only a couple of dysplastic nevi, but other people have more than 10. People who have dysplastic nevi usually also have an increased number of common moles.

Can a dysplastic nevus turn into melanoma?

Yes, but most dysplastic nevi do not turn into melanoma. Most remain stable over time. Researchers estimate that the chance of melanoma is about ten times greater for someone with more than five dysplastic nevi than for someone who has none, and the more dysplastic nevi a person has, the greater the chance of developing melanoma.

What should people do if they have a dysplastic nevus?

Everyone should protect their skin from the sun and stay away from sunlamps and tanning booths, but for people who have dysplastic nevi, it is even more important to protect the skin and avoid getting a suntan or sunburn. In addition, many doctors recommend that people with dysplastic nevi check their skin once a month. People should tell their doctor if they see any of the following changes in a dysplastic nevus:

- The color changes
- It gets smaller or bigger
- It changes in shape, texture, or height
- The skin on the surface becomes dry or scaly
- It becomes hard or feels lumpy
- It starts to itch
- It bleeds or oozes

Another thing that people with dysplastic nevi should do is get their skin examined by a doctor. Sometimes people or their doctors take photographs of dysplastic nevi so changes over time are easier to see. For people with many (more than five) dysplastic nevi, doctors may conduct a skin exam once or twice a year because of the moderately increased chance of melanoma. For people who also have a family history of melanoma, doctors may suggest a more frequent skin exam, such as every 3 to 6 months.

Should people have a doctor remove a dysplastic nevus or a common mole to prevent it from changing into melanoma?

No. Normally, people do not need to have a dysplastic nevus or common mole removed. One reason is that very few dysplastic nevi or common moles turn into melanoma. Another reason is that even removing all of the moles on the skin would not prevent the development of melanoma because melanoma can develop as a new colored area on the skin. That is why doctors usually remove only a mole that changes or a new colored area on the skin.

What is melanoma?

Melanoma is a type of skin cancer that begins in melanocytes. It is potentially dangerous because it can invade nearby tissues and spread to other parts of the body, such as the lung, liver, bone, or brain. The earlier that melanoma is detected and removed, the more likely that treatment will be successful.

Most melanocytes are in the skin, and melanoma can occur on any skin surface. It can develop from a common mole or dysplastic nevus, and it can also develop in an area of apparently normal skin. In addition, melanoma can also develop in the eye, the digestive tract, and other areas of the body.

When melanoma develops in men, it is often found on the head, neck, or back. When melanoma develops in women, it is often found on the back or on the lower legs.

People with dark skin are much less likely than people with fair skin to develop melanoma. When it does develop in people with dark skin, it is often found under the fingernails, under the toenails, on the palms of the hands, or on the soles of the feet.

What does melanoma look like?

Often the first sign of melanoma is a change in the shape, color, size, or feel of an existing mole. Melanoma may also appear as a new colored area on the skin.

The "ABCDE" rule describes the features of early melanoma:

- *Asymmetry*. The shape of one half does not match the other half.
- *Border that is irregular*. The edges are often ragged, notched, or blurred in outline. The pigment may spread into the surrounding skin.

- *Color that is uneven*. Shades of black, brown, and tan may be present. Areas of white, gray, red, pink, or blue may also be seen.
- *Diameter*. There is a change in size, usually an increase. Melanomas can be tiny, but most are larger than 6 millimeters wide (about 1/4 inch wide).
- *Evolving*. The mole has changed over the past few weeks or months.

Melanomas can vary greatly in how they look. Many show all of the ABCDE features. However, some may show only one or two of the ABCDE features.

In advanced melanoma, the texture of the mole may change. The skin on the surface may break down and look scraped. It may become hard or lumpy. The surface may ooze or bleed. Sometimes the melanoma is itchy, tender, or painful.

How is melanoma diagnosed?

The only way to diagnose melanoma is to remove tissue and check it for cancer cells. The doctor will remove all or part of the skin that looks abnormal. Usually, this procedure takes only a few minutes and can be done in a doctor's office, clinic, or hospital. The sample will be sent to a lab and a pathologist will look at the tissue under a microscope to check for melanoma.

What are the differences between a common mole, a dysplastic nevus, and a melanoma?

Common moles, dysplastic nevi, and melanoma vary by size, color, shape, and surface texture. The list below summarizes some differences between moles and cancer. Another important difference is that a common mole or dysplastic nevus will not return after it is removed by a full excisional biopsy from the skin, but melanoma sometimes grows back. Also, melanoma can spread to other parts of the body.

Common Mole (Nevus)

- *Is it cancer?* No. Common moles rarely become cancer.
- *How many people have common moles?* Most American adults—about 300 million people—have common moles.
- *How big are they?* Usually less than 5 millimeters wide, or about 1/4 inch (not as wide as a new pencil eraser).
- *What color are they?* May be pink, tan, brown, black (in people with dark skin), or a color that

is very close to a person's normal skin tone. The color is usually even throughout.

- *What shape are they?* Usually round or oval. A common mole has a distinct edge that separates it from the rest of the skin.
- *What is the surface texture?* Begins as a flat, smooth spot on the skin. May become raised and form a smooth bump.

Dysplastic Nevus

- *Is it cancer?* No. A dysplastic nevus is more likely than a common mole to become cancer, but most do not become cancer.
- *How many people have dysplastic nevi?* About 1 in 10 American adults—about 30 million people—have at least one dysplastic nevus.
- *How big are they?* Often wider than 5 millimeters (wider than a new pencil eraser).
- *What color are they?* May be a mixture of tan, brown, and red or pink shades.
- *What shape are they?* Have irregular or notched edges. May fade into the rest of the skin.
- *What is the surface texture?* May have a smooth, slightly scaly, or rough, irregular, and pebbly appearance.

Melanoma

- *Is it cancer?* Yes.

- *How many people have melanoma?* Melanoma is much less common than other kinds of skin cancer. But every year, about 2 in 10,000 Americans—more than 70,000 people—develop melanoma. More than 800,000 Americans alive today have been diagnosed with melanoma.

- *How big are they?* Usually wider than 6 millimeters (wider than a new pencil eraser).

- *What color are they?* Usually uneven in color. May have shades of black, brown, and tan. May also have areas of white, gray, red, pink, or blue.

- *What shape are they?* Often irregular and asymmetrical (the shape of one half does not match the other half). Edges may be ragged, notched, or blurred. May fade into the rest of the skin.

- *What is the surface texture?* May break down and look scraped, become hard or lumpy, or ooze or bleed.

What should people do if a mole changes, or they find a new mole or some other change on their skin?

People should tell their doctor if they find a new mole or a change in an existing mole. A family doctor may refer people with an unusual mole or other concerns about their skin to a dermatologist. A dermatologist is a doctor who specializes in diseases of the skin. Also, some plastic surgeons, general surgeons, internists, cancer specialists, and family doctors have special training in moles and melanoma.

What factors increase the change of melanoma?

People with the following risk factors have an increased chance of melanoma:

- *Having a dysplastic nevus*
- *Having more than 50 common moles*
- *Sunlight*: Sunlight is a source of UV radiation, which causes skin damage that can lead to melanoma and other skin cancers.
    - *Severe, blistering sunburns*: People who have had at least one severe, blistering sunburn have an increased chance of

melanoma. Although people who burn easily are more likely to have had sunburns as a child, sunburns during adulthood also increase the chance of melanoma.

- o *Lifetime sun exposure*: The greater the total amount of sun exposure over a lifetime, the greater the chance of melanoma.

- o *Tanning*: Although having skin that tans well lowers the risk of sunburn, even people who tan well without sunburning increase their chance of melanoma by spending time in the sun without protection.

Sunlight can be reflected by sand, water, snow, ice, and pavement. The sun's rays can get through clouds, windshields, windows, and light clothing.

In the United States, skin cancer is more common where the sun is strong. For example, a larger proportion of people in Texas than Minnesota get skin cancer. Also, the sun is strong at higher elevations, such as in the mountains.

- *Sunlamps and tanning booths*: UV radiation from artificial sources, such as sunlamps and tanning booths, can cause skin damage and melanoma. Health care providers strongly encourage people, especially young people, to avoid using sunlamps and tanning booths. The risk of skin cancer is greatly increased by using sunlamps and tanning booths before age 30.

- *Personal history*: People who have had melanoma have an increased risk of developing other melanomas.

- *Family history*: Melanoma sometimes runs in families. People who have two or more close relatives (mother, father, sister, brother, or child) with melanoma have an increased chance of melanoma. In rare cases, members of a family will have an inherited disorder, such as xeroderma pigmentosum, that makes the skin extremely sensitive to the sun and greatly increases the chance of melanoma.

- *Skin that burns easily*: People who have fair (pale) skin that burns easily in the sun, blue or

gray eyes, red or blond hair, or many freckles
have an increased chance of melanoma.

- *Certain medical conditions or medicines*:
  Medical conditions or medicines (such as some
  antibiotics, hormones, or antidepressants) that
  make skin more sensitive to the sun or that
  suppress the immune system increase the chance
  of melanoma.

How can people protect their skin from the sun?

The best way to prevent melanoma is to limit exposure to
sunlight. Having a suntan or sunburn means that the skin
has been damaged by the sun, and continued tanning or
burning increases the chance of developing melanoma.

Chapter 18: Fluoridated Water and Cancer Risk

- Fluoride in water helps to prevent and can even reverse tooth decay.
- More than 60 percent of the U.S. population has access to fluoridated water through public water supply systems.
- The optimal level of fluoride to prevent tooth decay is 0.7 milligrams per liter of water.
- Many studies, in both humans and animals, have shown no association between fluoridated water and cancer risk.

What is fluoride, and where is it found?

Fluoride is the name given to a group of compounds that are composed of the naturally occurring element fluorine and one or more other elements. Fluorides are present naturally in water and soil at varying levels.

In the 1940s, scientists discovered that people who lived where drinking water supplies had naturally occurring fluoride levels of approximately 1 part fluoride per million parts water or greater (>1.0 ppm) had fewer dental caries (cavities) than people who lived where fluoride levels in drinking water were lower. Many more recent studies have supported this finding.

It was subsequently found that fluoride can prevent and even reverse tooth decay by inhibiting bacteria that produce acid in the mouth and by enhancing remineralization, the process through which tooth enamel is "rebuilt" after it begins to decay.

In addition to building up in teeth, ingested fluoride accumulates in bones.

What is water fluoridation?

Water fluoridation is the process of adding fluoride to the water supply so the level reaches approximately 0.7 ppm, or 0.7 milligrams of fluoride per liter of water; this is the optimal level for preventing tooth decay.

Can fluoridated water cause cancer?

A possible relationship between fluoridated water and cancer risk has been debated for years. The debate resurfaced in 1990 when a study by the National Toxicology Program, part of the National Institute of Environmental Health Sciences, showed an increased number of osteosarcomas (bone tumors) in male rats given water high in fluoride for 2 years. However, other studies in humans and in animals have not shown an association between fluoridated water and cancer.

In a February 1991 Public Health Service (PHS) report, the agency said it found no evidence of an association between fluoride and cancer in humans. The report, based on a review of more than 50 human epidemiological (population) studies produced over the past 40 years, concluded that optimal fluoridation of drinking water "does not pose a detectable cancer risk to humans" as evidenced by extensive human epidemiological data reported to date. In one of the studies reviewed for the PHS report, scientists at NCI evaluated the relationship between the fluoridation of drinking water and the number of deaths due to cancer in the United States during a 36-year period, and the relationship between water fluoridation and number of new cases of cancer during a 15-year period. After examining more than 2.2 million cancer death records and 125,000 cancer case records in counties using fluoridated water, the researchers found no indication of increased cancer risk associated with fluoridated drinking water.

In 1993, the Subcommittee on Health Effects of Ingested Fluoride of the National Research Council, part of the National Academy of Sciences, conducted an extensive literature review concerning the association between fluoridated drinking water and increased cancer risk. The review included data from more than 50 human epidemiological studies and six animal studies. The Subcommittee concluded that none of the data demonstrated an association between fluoridated drinking water and cancer. A 1999 report by the CDC supported these findings. The CDC report concluded that studies to date have produced "no credible evidence" of an association between fluoridated drinking water and an increased risk for cancer. Subsequent interview studies of patients with osteosarcoma and their parents produced conflicting results, but with none showing clear evidence of a causal relationship between fluoride intake and risk of this tumor.

Recently, researchers examined the possible relationship between fluoride exposure and osteosarcoma in a new way: they measured fluoride concentration in samples of normal bone that were adjacent to a person's tumor. Because fluoride naturally accumulates in bone, this method provides a more accurate measure of cumulative fluoride exposure than relying on the memory of study participants or municipal water treatment records. The analysis showed no difference in bone fluoride levels between people with osteosarcoma and people in a control group who had other malignant bone tumors.

Chapter 19: Genetic Testing for Hereditary Cancer Syndromes

- Genetic mutations play a role in the development of all cancers. Most of these mutations occur during a person's lifetime, but some mutations, including those that are associated with hereditary cancer syndromes, can be inherited from a person's parents.
- Inherited mutations play a major role in the development of about 5 to 10 percent of all cancers.
- The genetic mutations associated with more than 50 hereditary cancer syndromes have been identified, and genetic tests can help tell whether a person from a family with such a syndrome has one of these mutations.
- A genetic counselor, doctor, or other health care professional trained in genetics can help an individual or family understand genetic test results.

What is genetic testing?

Genetic testing looks for specific inherited changes (mutations) in a person's chromosomes, genes, or proteins. Genetic mutations can have harmful, beneficial, neutral (no effect), or uncertain effects on health. Mutations that are harmful may increase a person's chance, or risk, of developing a disease such as cancer. Overall, inherited mutations are thought to play a role in about 5 to 10 percent of all cancers.

Cancer can sometimes appear to "run in families" even if it is not caused by an inherited mutation. For example, a shared environment or lifestyle, such as tobacco use, can cause similar cancers to develop among family members. However, certain patterns—such as the types of cancer that develop, other non-cancer conditions that are seen, and the ages at which cancer typically develops—may suggest the presence of a hereditary cancer syndrome.

The genetic mutations that cause many of the known hereditary cancer syndromes have been identified, and genetic testing can confirm whether a condition is, indeed, the result of an inherited syndrome. Genetic testing is also done to determine whether family members without obvious illness have inherited the same mutation as a family member who is known to carry a cancer-associated mutation.

Inherited genetic mutations can increase a person's risk of developing cancer through a variety of mechanisms, depending on the function of the gene. Mutations in genes that control cell growth and the repair of damaged DNA are particularly likely to be associated with increased cancer risk.

Genetic testing of tumor samples can also be performed, but this Fact Sheet does not cover such testing.

Does someone who inherits a cancer-predisposing mutation always get cancer?

No. Even if a cancer-predisposing mutation is present in a family, it does not necessarily mean that everyone who inherits the mutation will develop cancer. Several factors influence the outcome in a given person with the mutation. One factor is the pattern of inheritance of the cancer syndrome. To understand how hereditary cancer syndromes may be inherited, it is helpful to keep in mind that every person has two copies of most genes, with one copy inherited from each parent. Most mutations involved in hereditary cancer syndromes are inherited in one of two main patterns: autosomal dominant and autosomal recessive.

With autosomal dominant inheritance, a single altered copy of the gene is enough to increase a person's chances of developing cancer. In this case, the parent from whom the mutation was inherited may also show the effects of the gene mutation. The parent may also be referred to as a carrier.

With autosomal recessive inheritance, a person has an increased risk of cancer only if he or she inherits a mutant (altered) copy of the gene from each parent. The parents, who each carry one copy of the altered gene along with a normal (unaltered) copy, do not usually have an increased risk of cancer themselves. However, because they can pass the altered gene to their children, they are called carriers.

A third form of inheritance of cancer-predisposing mutations is X-linked recessive inheritance. Males have a single X chromosome, which they inherit from their mothers, and females have two X chromosomes (one from each parent). A female with a recessive cancer-predisposing mutation on one of her X chromosomes and a normal copy of the gene on her other X chromosome is a carrier but will not have an increased risk of cancer. Her sons, however, will have only the altered copy of the gene and will therefore have an increased risk of cancer.

Even when people have one copy of a dominant cancer-predisposing mutation, two copies of a recessive mutation, or, for males, one copy of an X-linked recessive mutation, they may not develop cancer. Some mutations are "incompletely penetrant," which means that only some people will show the effects of these mutations. Mutations can also "vary in their expressivity," which means that the severity of the symptoms may vary from person to person.

What genetic tests are available for cancer risk?

More than 50 hereditary cancer syndromes have been described. The majority of these are caused by highly penetrant mutations that are inherited in a dominant fashion. The list below includes some of the more common inherited cancer syndromes for which genetic testing is available, the gene(s) that are mutated in each syndrome, and the cancer types most often associated with these syndromes.

Hereditary breast cancer and ovarian cancer syndrome

- Genes: BRCA1, BRCA2
- Related cancer types: Female breast, ovarian, and other cancers, including prostate, pancreatic, and male breast cancer

Li-Fraumeni syndrome

- Gene: TP53
- Related cancer types: Breast cancer, soft tissue sarcoma, osteosarcoma (bone cancer), leukemia, brain tumors, adrenocortical carcinoma (cancer of the adrenal glands), and other cancers

Cowden syndrome (PTEN hamartoma tumor syndrome)

- Gene: PTEN
- Related cancer types: Breast, thyroid, endometrial (uterine lining), and other cancers

Lynch syndrome (hereditary nonpolyposis colorectal cancer)

- Genes: MSH2, MLH1, MSH6, PMS2, EPCAM
- Related cancer types: Colorectal, endometrial, ovarian, renal pelvis, pancreatic, small intestine, liver and biliary tract, stomach, brain, and breast cancers

Familial adenomatous polyposis

- Gene: APC
- Related cancer types: Colorectal cancer, multiple non-malignant colon polyps, and both non-cancerous (benign) and cancerous tumors in the small intestine, brain, stomach, bone, skin, and other tissues

Retinoblastoma

- Gene: RB1
- Related cancer types: Eye cancer (cancer of the retina), pinealoma (cancer of the pineal gland), osteosarcoma, melanoma, and soft tissue sarcoma

Multiple endocrine neoplasia type 1 (Wermer syndrome)

- Gene: MEN1
- Related cancer types: Pancreatic endocrine tumors and (usually benign) parathyroid and pituitary gland tumors

Multiple endocrine neoplasia type 2

- Gene: RET
- Related cancer types: Medullary thyroid cancer and pheochromocytoma (benign adrenal gland tumor)

Von Hippel-Lindau syndrome

- Gene: VHL
- Related cancer types: Kidney cancer and multiple noncancerous tumors, including pheochromocytoma

Who should consider genetic testing for cancer risk?

Many experts recommend that genetic testing for cancer risk should be strongly considered when all three of the following criteria are met:

- The person being tested has a personal or family history that suggests an inherited cancer risk condition
- The test results can be adequately interpreted (that is, they can clearly tell whether a specific genetic change is present or absent)
- The results provide information that will help guide a person's future medical care

The features of a person's personal or family medical history that, particularly in combination, may suggest a hereditary cancer syndrome include:

- Cancer that was diagnosed at an unusually young age
- Several different types of cancer that have occurred independently in the same person
- Cancer that has developed in both organs in a set of paired organs, such as both kidneys or both breasts
- Several close blood relatives that have the same type of cancer (for example, a mother, daughter, and sisters with breast cancer)

- Unusual cases of a specific cancer type (for example, breast cancer in a man)
- The presence of birth defects, such as certain noncancerous (benign) skin growths or skeletal abnormalities, that are known to be associated with inherited cancer syndromes
- Being a member of a racial/ethnic group that is known to have an increased chance of having a certain hereditary cancer syndrome and having one or more of the above features as well

It is strongly recommended that a person who is considering genetic testing speak with a professional trained in genetics before deciding whether to be tested. These professionals can include doctors, genetic counselors, and other health care providers (such as nurses, psychologists, or social workers). Genetic counseling can help people consider the risks, benefits, and limitations of genetic testing in their particular situation. Sometimes the genetic professional finds that testing is not needed. Genetic counseling includes a detailed review of the individual's personal and family medical history related to possible cancer risk. Counseling also includes discussions about such issues as:

- Whether genetic testing is appropriate, which specific test(s) might be used, and the technical accuracy of the test(s)
- The medical implications of a positive or a negative test result (see below)
- The possibility that a test result might not be informative—that is, that the information may not be useful in making health care decisions (see below)
- The psychological risks and benefits of learning one's genetic test results
- The risk of passing a genetic mutation (if one is present in a parent) to children

Learning about these issues is a key part of the informed consent process. Written informed consent is strongly recommended before a genetic test is ordered. People give their consent by signing a form saying that they have been told about, and understand, the purpose of the test, its medical implications, the risks and benefits of the test, possible alternatives to the test, and their privacy rights. Unlike most other medical tests, genetic tests can reveal information not only about the person being tested but also about that person's relatives. The presence of a harmful genetic mutation in one family member makes it more likely that other blood relatives may also carry the same mutation. Family relationships can be affected when one member of a family discloses genetic test results that may have implications for other family members. Family members may have very different opinions about how useful it is to learn whether they do or do not have a disease-related genetic mutation. Health discussions may get complicated when some family members know their genetic status while other family members do not choose to know their test results. A conversation with genetics professionals may help family members better understand the complicated choices they may face.

How is genetic testing done?

Genetic tests are usually requested by a person's doctor or other health care provider. Although it may be possible to obtain some genetic tests without a health care provider's order, this approach is not recommended because it does not give the patient the valuable opportunity to discuss this complicated decision with a knowledgeable professional. Testing is done on a small sample of body fluid or tissue—usually blood, but sometimes saliva, cells from inside the cheek, skin cells, or amniotic fluid (the fluid surrounding a developing fetus).

The sample is then sent to a laboratory that specializes in genetic testing. The laboratory returns the test results to the doctor or genetic counselor who requested the test. In some cases, the laboratory may send the results to the patient directly. It usually takes several weeks or longer to get the test results. Genetic counseling is recommended both before and after genetic testing to make sure that patients have accurate information about what a particular genetic test means for their health and care.

What do the results of genetic testing mean?

Genetic testing can have several possible results: positive, negative, true negative, uninformative negative, false negative, variant of unknown significance, or benign polymorphism. These results are described below.

A "positive test result" means that the laboratory found a specific genetic alteration (or mutation) that is associated with a hereditary cancer syndrome. A positive result may:

- Confirm the diagnosis of a hereditary cancer syndrome
- Indicate an increased risk of developing certain cancer(s) in the future
- Show that someone carries a particular genetic change that does not increase their own risk of

cancer but that may increase the risk in their children if they also inherit an altered copy from their other parent (that is, if the child inherits two copies of the abnormal gene, one from their mother and one from their father).

- Suggest a need for further testing
- Provide important information that can help other family members make decisions about their own health care.

Also, people who have a positive test result that indicates that they have an increased risk of developing cancer in the future may be able to take steps to lower their risk of developing cancer or to find cancer earlier, including:

- Being checked at a younger age or more often for signs of cancer
- Reducing their cancer risk by taking medications or having surgery to remove "at-risk" tissue (These approaches to risk reduction are options for only a few inherited cancer syndromes.)
- Changing personal behaviors (like quitting smoking, getting more exercise, and eating a healthier diet) to reduce the risk of certain cancers

A positive result on a prenatal genetic test for cancer risk may influence a decision about whether to continue a pregnancy. The results of pre-implantation testing (performed on embryos created by in vitro fertilization) can guide a doctor in deciding which embryo (or embryos) to implant in a woman's uterus.

Finally, in patients who have already been diagnosed with cancer, a positive result for a mutation associated with certain hereditary cancer syndromes can influence how the cancer is treated. For example, some hereditary cancer disorders interfere with the body's ability to repair damage that occurs to cellular DNA. If someone with one of these conditions receives a standard dose of radiation or chemotherapy to treat their cancer, they may experience severe, potentially life-threatening treatment side effects. Knowing about the genetic disorder before treatment begins allows doctors to modify the treatment and reduce the severity of the side effects.

A "negative test result" means that the laboratory did not find the specific alteration that the test was designed to detect. This result is most useful when working with a family in which the specific, disease-causing genetic alteration is already known to be present. In such a case, a negative result can show that the tested family member has not inherited the mutation that is present in their family and that this person therefore does not have the inherited cancer syndrome tested for, does not have an increased genetic risk of developing cancer, or is not a carrier of a mutation that increases cancer risk. Such a test result is called a "true negative." A true negative result does not mean that there is no cancer risk, but rather that the risk is probably the same as the cancer risk in the general population.

When a person has a strong family history of cancer but the family has not been found to have a known mutation associated with a hereditary cancer syndrome, a negative test result is classified as an "uninformative negative" (that is, does not provide useful information). It is not possible to tell whether someone has a harmful gene mutation that was not detected by the particular test used (a "false negative") or whether the person truly has no cancer-predisposing genetic alterations in that gene. It is also possible for a person to have a mutation in a gene other than the gene that was tested.

If genetic testing shows a change that has not been previously associated with cancer in other people, the person's test result may report "variant of unknown significance," or VUS. This result may be interpreted as "ambiguous" (uncertain), which is to say that the information does not help in making health care decisions. If the test reveals a genetic change that is common in the general population among people without cancer, the change is called a polymorphism. Everyone has commonly occurring genetic variations (polymorphisms) that are not associated with any increased risk of disease.

Chapter 20: BRCA1 and BRCA2: Cancer Risk and Genetic Testing

- BRCA1 and BRCA2 are human genes that belong to a class of genes known as tumor suppressors. Mutation of these genes has been linked to hereditary breast and ovarian cancer.

- A woman's risk of developing breast and/or ovarian cancer is greatly increased if she inherits a deleterious (harmful) BRCA1 or BRCA2 mutation. Men with these mutations also have an increased risk of breast cancer. Both men and women who have harmful BRCA1 or BRCA2 mutations may be at increased risk of other cancers.

- Genetic tests are available to check for BRCA1 and BRCA2 mutations. A blood sample is required for these tests, and genetic counseling is recommended before and after the tests.

- If a harmful BRCA1 or BRCA2 mutation is found, several options are available to help a person manage their cancer risk.

- Federal and state laws help ensure the privacy of a person's genetic information and provide protection against discrimination in health insurance and employment practices.

- Many research studies are being conducted to find newer and better ways of detecting, treating, and preventing cancer in BRCA1 and BRCA2 mutation carriers. Additional studies are focused on improving genetic counseling methods and outcomes. Our knowledge in these areas is evolving rapidly.

What are BRCA1 and BRCA2?

BRCA1 and BRCA2 are human genes that belong to a class of genes known as tumor suppressors.

In normal cells, BRCA1 and BRCA2 help ensure the stability of the cell's genetic material (DNA) and help prevent uncontrolled cell growth. Mutation of these genes has been linked to the development of hereditary breast and ovarian cancer.

The names BRCA1 and BRCA2 stand for **b**reast **c**ancer susceptibility gene **1** and **b**reast **c**ancer susceptibility gene **2**, respectively.

How do BRCA1 and BRCA2 gene mutations affect a person's risk of cancer?

Not all gene changes, or mutations, are deleterious (harmful). Some mutations may be beneficial, whereas others may have no obvious effect (neutral). Harmful mutations can increase a person's risk of developing a disease, such as cancer.

A woman's lifetime risk of developing breast and/or ovarian cancer is greatly increased if she inherits a harmful mutation in BRCA1 or BRCA2. Such a woman has an increased risk of developing breast and/or ovarian cancer at an early age (before menopause) and often has multiple, close family members who have been diagnosed with these diseases. Harmful BRCA1 mutations may also increase a woman's risk of developing cervical, uterine, pancreatic, and colon cancer. Harmful BRCA2 mutations may additionally increase the risk of pancreatic cancer, stomach cancer, gallbladder and bile duct cancer, and melanoma. Men with harmful BRCA1 mutations also have an increased risk of breast cancer and, possibly, of pancreatic cancer, testicular cancer, and early-onset prostate cancer. However, male breast cancer, pancreatic cancer, and prostate cancer appear to be more strongly associated with BRCA2 gene mutations.

The likelihood that a breast and/or ovarian cancer is associated with a harmful mutation in BRCA1 or BRCA2 is highest in families with a history of multiple cases of breast cancer, cases of both breast and ovarian cancer, one or more family members with two primary cancers (original tumors that develop at different sites in the body), or an Ashkenazi (Central and Eastern European) Jewish background. However, not every woman in such families carries a harmful BRCA1 or BRCA2 mutation, and not every cancer in such families is linked to a harmful mutation in one of these genes. Furthermore, not every woman who has a harmful BRCA1 or BRCA2 mutation will develop breast and/or ovarian cancer.

According to estimates of lifetime risk, about 12.0 percent of women (120 out of 1,000) in the general population will develop breast cancer sometime during their lives compared with about 60 percent of women (600 out of 1,000) who have inherited a harmful mutation in BRCA1 or BRCA2. In other words, a woman who has inherited a harmful mutation in BRCA1 or BRCA2 is about five times more likely to develop breast cancer than a woman who does not have such a mutation.

Lifetime risk estimates for ovarian cancer among women in the general population indicate that 1.4 percent (14 out of 1,000) will be diagnosed with ovarian cancer compared with 15 to 40 percent of women (150–400 out of 1,000) who have a harmful BRCA1 or BRCA2 mutation.

It is important to note, however, that most research related to BRCA1 and BRCA2 has been done on large families with many individuals affected by cancer. Estimates of breast and ovarian cancer risk associated with BRCA1 and BRCA2 mutations have been calculated from studies of these families. Because family members share a proportion of their genes and, often, their environment, it is possible that the large number of cancer cases seen in these families may be due in part to other genetic or environmental factors. Therefore, risk estimates that are based on families with many affected members may not accurately reflect the levels of risk for BRCA1 and BRCA2 mutation carriers in the general population. In addition, no data are available from long-term studies of the general population comparing cancer risk in women who have harmful BRCA1 or BRCA2 mutations with women who do not have such mutations. Therefore, the percentages given above are estimates that may change as more data become available.

Do inherited mutations in other genes increase the risk of breast and/or ovarian tumors?

Yes. Mutations in several other genes, including TP53, PTEN, STK11/LKB1, CDH1, CHEK2, ATM, MLH1, and MSH2, have been associated with hereditary breast and/or ovarian tumors. However, the majority of hereditary breast cancers can be accounted for by inherited mutations in BRCA1 and BRCA2. Overall, it has been estimated that inherited BRCA1 and BRCA2 mutations account for 5 to 10 percent of breast cancers and 10 to 15 percent of ovarian cancers among white women in the United States.

Are specific mutations in BRCA1 and BRCA2 more common in certain populations?

Yes. For example, three specific mutations, two in the BRCA1 gene and one in the BRCA2 gene, are the most common mutations found in these genes in the Ashkenazi Jewish population. In one study, 2.3 percent of participants (120 out of 5,318) carried one of these three mutations. This frequency is about five times higher than that found in the general population. It is not known whether the increased frequency of these mutations is responsible for the increased risk of breast cancer in Jewish populations compared with non-Jewish populations.

Other ethnic and geographic populations around the world, such as the Norwegian, Dutch, and Icelandic peoples, also have higher frequencies of specific BRCA1 and BRCA2 mutations.

In addition, limited data indicate that the frequencies of specific BRCA1 and BRCA2 mutations may vary among individual racial and ethnic groups in the United States, including African Americans, Hispanics, Asian Americans, and non-Hispanic whites.

This information about genetic differences between racial and ethnic groups may help health care providers in selecting the most appropriate genetic test(s).

Are genetic tests available to detect BRCA1 and BRCA2 mutations, and how are they performed?

Yes. Several methods are available to test for BRCA1 and BRCA2 mutations. Most of these methods look for changes in BRCA1 and BRCA2 DNA. At least one method looks for changes in the proteins produced by these genes. Frequently, a combination of methods is used.

A blood sample is needed for these tests. The blood is drawn in a laboratory, doctor's office, hospital, or clinic and then sent to a laboratory that specializes in the tests. It usually takes several weeks or longer to get the test results. Individuals who decide to get tested should check with their health care provider to find out when their test results might be available.

Genetic counseling is generally recommended before and after a genetic test. This counseling should be performed by a health care professional who is experienced in cancer genetics. Genetic counseling usually involves a risk assessment based on the individual's personal and family medical history and discussions about the appropriateness of genetic testing, the specific test(s) that might be used and the technical accuracy of the test(s), the medical implications of a positive or a negative test result, the possibility that a test result might not be informative (an ambiguous result), the psychological risks and benefits of genetic test results, and the risk of passing a mutation to children.

How do people know if they should consider genetic testing for BRCA1 and BRCA2 mutations?

Currently, there are no standard criteria for recommending or referring someone for BRCA1 or BRCA2 mutation testing.

In a family with a history of breast and/or ovarian cancer, it may be most informative to first test a family member who has breast or ovarian cancer. If that person is found to have a harmful BRCA1 or BRCA2 mutation, then other family members can be tested to see if they also have the mutation. Regardless, women who have a relative with a harmful BRCA1 or BRCA2 mutation and women who appear to be at increased risk of breast and/or ovarian cancer because of their family history should consider genetic counseling to learn more about their potential risks and about BRCA1 and BRCA2 genetic tests.

The likelihood of a harmful mutation in BRCA1 or BRCA2 is increased with certain familial patterns of cancer. These patterns include the following:

- For women who are not of Ashkenazi Jewish descent:
  o two first-degree relatives (mother, daughter, or sister) diagnosed with breast cancer, one of whom was diagnosed at age 50 or younger;
  o three or more first-degree or second-degree (grandmother or aunt) relatives diagnosed with breast cancer regardless of their age at diagnosis;
  o a combination of first- and second-degree relatives diagnosed with breast

cancer and ovarian cancer (one cancer type per person);

- o a first-degree relative with cancer diagnosed in both breasts (bilateral breast cancer);
- o a combination of two or more first- or second-degree relatives diagnosed with ovarian cancer regardless of age at diagnosis;
- o a first- or second-degree relative diagnosed with both breast and ovarian cancer regardless of age at diagnosis; and
- o breast cancer diagnosed in a male relative.

- For women of Ashkenazi Jewish descent:
  - o any first-degree relative diagnosed with breast or ovarian cancer; and
  - o two second-degree relatives on the same side of the family diagnosed with breast or ovarian cancer.

These family history patterns apply to about 2 percent of adult women in the general population. Women who have none of these family history patterns have a low probability of having a harmful BRCA1 or BRCA2 mutation.

What does a positive BRCA1 or BRCA2 test result mean?

A positive test result generally indicates that a person has inherited a known harmful mutation in BRCA1 or BRCA2 and, therefore, has an increased risk of developing certain cancers, as described above. However, a positive test result provides information only about a person's risk of developing cancer. It cannot tell whether an individual will actually develop cancer or when. Not all women who inherit a harmful BRCA1 or BRCA2 mutation will develop breast or ovarian cancer.

A positive genetic test result may have important health and social implications for family members, including future generations. Unlike most other medical tests, genetic tests can reveal information not only about the person being tested but also about that person's relatives. Both men and women who inherit harmful BRCA1 or BRCA2 mutations, whether they develop cancer themselves or not, may pass the mutations on to their sons and daughters. However, not all children of people who have a harmful mutation will inherit the mutation.

What does a negative BRCA1 or BRCA2 test result mean?

How a negative test result will be interpreted depends on whether or not someone in the tested person's family is known to carry a harmful BRCA1 or BRCA2 mutation. If someone in the family has a known mutation, testing other family members for the same mutation can provide information about their cancer risk. If a person tests negative for a known mutation in his or her family, it is unlikely that they have an inherited susceptibility to cancer associated with BRCA1 or BRCA2. Such a test result is called a "true negative." Having a true negative test result does not mean that a person will not develop cancer; it means that the person's risk of cancer is probably the same as that of people in the general population.

In cases in which a family has a history of breast and/or ovarian cancer and no known mutation in BRCA1 or BRCA2 has been previously identified, a negative test result is not informative. It is not possible to tell whether an individual has a harmful BRCA1 or BRCA2 mutation that was not detected by testing (a "false negative") or whether the result is a true negative. In addition, it is possible for people to have a mutation in a gene other than BRCA1 or

BRCA2 that increases their cancer risk but is not detectable by the test(s) used.

What does an ambiguous BRCA1 or BRCA2 test result mean?

If genetic testing shows a change in BRCA1 or BRCA2 that has not been previously associated with cancer in other people, the person's test result may be interpreted as "ambiguous" (uncertain). One study found that 10 percent of women who underwent BRCA1 and BRCA2 mutation testing had this type of ambiguous result.

Because everyone has genetic differences that are not associated with an increased risk of disease, it is sometimes not known whether a specific DNA change affects a person's risk of developing cancer. As more research is conducted and more people are tested for BRCA1 or BRCA2 changes, scientists will learn more about these changes and cancer risk.

What are the options for a person who has a positive test result?

Several options are available for managing cancer risk in individuals who have a harmful BRCA1 or BRCA2 mutation. However, high-quality data on the effectiveness of these options are limited.

- *Surveillance*—Surveillance means cancer screening, or a way of detecting the disease early. Screening does not, however, change the risk of developing cancer. The goal is to find cancer early, when it may be most treatable. Surveillance methods for breast cancer may include mammography and clinical breast exams. Studies are currently under way to test the effectiveness of other breast cancer screening methods, such as magnetic resonance imaging (MRI), in women with BRCA1 or BRCA2 mutations. With careful surveillance, many breast cancers will be diagnosed early enough to be successfully treated.

  For ovarian cancer, surveillance methods may include transvaginal ultrasound, blood tests for CA–125 antigen, and clinical exams. Surveillance can sometimes find ovarian cancer at an early stage, but it is uncertain whether these methods can help reduce a woman's chance of dying from this disease.

- *Prophylactic Surgery*—This type of surgery involves removing as much of the "at-risk" tissue as possible in order to reduce the chance of developing cancer. Bilateral prophylactic mastectomy (removal of healthy breasts) and prophylactic salpingo-oophorectomy (removal of healthy fallopian tubes and ovaries) do not, however, offer a guarantee against developing cancer. Because not all at-risk tissue can be removed by these procedures, some women have developed breast cancer, ovarian cancer, or primary peritoneal carcinomatosis (a type of cancer similar to ovarian cancer) even after prophylactic surgery. In addition, some evidence suggests that the amount of protection salpingo-oophorectomy provides against the development of breast and ovarian cancer may differ between carriers of BRCA1 and BRCA2 mutations.

- *Risk Avoidance*—Certain behaviors have been associated with breast and ovarian cancer risk in the general population. Research results on the benefits of modifying individual behaviors to reduce the risk of developing cancer among

BRCA1 or BRCA2 mutation carriers are limited.

- *Chemoprevention*—This approach involves the use of natural or synthetic substances to reduce the risk of developing cancer or to reduce the chance that cancer will come back. For example, the drug tamoxifen has been shown in numerous clinical studies to reduce the risk of developing breast cancer by about 50 percent in women who are at increased risk of this disease and to reduce the recurrence of breast cancer in women undergoing treatment for a previously diagnosed breast tumor. As a result, tamoxifen was approved by the U.S. Food and Drug Administration (FDA) as a breast cancer treatment and to reduce the risk of breast cancer development in premenopausal and postmenopausal women who are at increased risk of this disease. Few studies, however, have evaluated the effectiveness of tamoxifen in women with BRCA1 or BRCA2 mutations. Data from three studies suggest that tamoxifen may be able to help lower the risk of breast cancer in BRCA1 and BRCA2 mutation carriers. Two of these studies examined the effectiveness of tamoxifen in helping to reduce the development of cancer in the opposite breast of women undergoing treatment for an initial breast cancer.

Another drug, raloxifene, was shown in a large clinical trial sponsored by the National Cancer Institute (NCI) to reduce the risk of developing invasive breast cancer in postmenopausal women at increased risk of this disease by about the same amount as tamoxifen. As a result, raloxifene was approved by the FDA for breast cancer risk reduction in postmenopausal women. Since tamoxifen and raloxifene inhibit the growth of breast cancer cells in similar ways, raloxifene may be able to help reduce breast cancer risk in postmenopausal BRCA1 and BRCA2 mutation carriers. However, this has not been studied directly.

What are some of the benefits of genetic testing for breast and ovarian cancer risk?

There can be benefits to genetic testing, whether a person receives a positive or a negative result. The potential benefits of a negative result include a sense of relief and the possibility that special preventive checkups, tests, or surgeries may not be needed. A positive test result can bring relief from uncertainty and allow people to make informed decisions about their future, including taking steps to reduce their cancer risk. In addition, many people who have a positive test result may be able to participate in medical research that could, in the long run, help reduce deaths from breast cancer.

What are some of the risks of genetic testing for breast and ovarian cancer risk?

The direct medical risks, or harms, of genetic testing are very small, but test results may have an effect on a person's emotions, social relationships, finances, and medical choices.

People who receive a positive test result may feel anxious, depressed, or angry. They may choose to undergo preventive measures, such as prophylactic surgery, that have serious long-term implications and whose effectiveness is uncertain.

People who receive a negative test result may experience "survivor guilt," caused by the knowledge that they likely do not have an increased risk of developing a disease that affects one or more loved ones.

Because genetic testing can reveal information about more than one family member, the emotions caused by test results can create tension within families. Test results can also affect personal choices, such as marriage and childbearing. Issues surrounding the privacy and confidentiality of genetic test results are additional potential risks

In general, what factors increase or decrease the chance of developing breast cancer and/or ovarian cancer?

The following factors have been associated with increased or decreased risk of developing breast and/or ovarian cancer in the general population. It is not yet known exactly how these factors influence risk in people with BRCA1 or BRCA2 mutations. In addition, a significant portion of hereditary breast cancers are not associated with BRCA1 or BRCA2 mutations.

- *Age*—The risks of breast and ovarian cancer increase with age. Most breast and ovarian cancers occur in women over the age of 50. Women with harmful BRCA1 or BRCA2 mutations often develop breast or ovarian cancer before age 50.

- *Family History*—Women who have a first-degree relative (mother, sister, or daughter) or other close relative with breast and/or ovarian cancer may be at increased risk of developing these cancers. In addition, women with relatives who have had colon cancer may be at increased risk of developing ovarian cancer.

- *Medical History*—Women who have already had breast cancer are at increased risk of developing breast cancer again, or of developing ovarian cancer.

- *Hormonal Influences*—Estrogen is a hormone that is naturally produced by the body and stimulates the normal growth of breast tissue. It is thought that excess estrogen may contribute to breast cancer risk because of its natural role in stimulating breast cell growth. Women who had their first menstrual period before the age of 12 or experienced menopause after age 55 have a slightly increased risk of breast cancer, as do women who had their first child after age 30. Each of these factors increases the amount of time a woman's body is exposed to estrogen. Removal of a woman's ovaries, which are the main source of estrogen production, reduces the risk of breast cancer. Breast-feeding also reduces breast cancer risk and is thought to exert its effects through hormonal mechanisms.

- *Birth Control Pills (Oral Contraceptives)*— Most studies have shown a slight increase or no change in risk of breast cancer among women taking birth control pills. In contrast, numerous studies have shown that taking birth control pills decreases a woman's risk of developing ovarian cancer. This protective benefit appears to increase with the duration of oral contraceptive use and persists up to 25 years after discontinuing use. It also appears that the use of birth control pills lowers the risk of ovarian cancer in women who carry harmful BRCA1 or BRCA2 mutations.

- *Hormone Replacement Therapy*—Doctors may prescribe hormone replacement therapy (HRT) to reduce the discomfort of certain symptoms of menopause, such as hot flashes. However, the results of the Women's Health Initiative (WHI), a large clinical study conducted by the National Heart, Lung, and Blood Institute, part of the National Institutes of Health (NIH), showed that HRT with the hormones estrogen and progestin is associated with harmful side effects, including an increased risk of breast cancer and increased risks of heart attack, blood clots, and stroke. The WHI also showed that HRT with estrogen alone was associated with increased risks of blood clots and stroke, but the effect on breast cancer risk was uncertain. In addition, the WHI showed an increase in ovarian cancer risk among women who received estrogen and progestin HRT, but this finding was not statistically significant. Because of these potential harmful side effects, the FDA has recommended that HRT be used only at the lowest doses for the shortest period of time needed to achieve treatment goals.

No data have been reported to date regarding the effects of HRT on breast cancer risk among women carrying harmful BRCA1 or BRCA2 mutations, and only limited data are available regarding HRT use and ovarian cancer risk among such women. In one study, HRT use did not appear to affect ovarian cancer risk among women with BRCA1 or BRCA2 mutations. When considering HRT use, both the potential harms and benefits of this type of treatment should be discussed carefully by a woman and her health care provider.

- *Obesity*—Substantial evidence indicates that obesity is associated with an increased risk of breast cancer, especially among postmenopausal women who have not used HRT. Evidence also suggests that obesity is associated with increased mortality (death) from ovarian cancer.

- *Physical Activity*—Numerous studies have examined the relationship between physical activity and breast cancer risk, and most of these studies have shown that physical activity, especially strenuous physical activity, is associated with reduced risk. This decrease in risk appears to be more pronounced in premenopausal women and women with lower-than-normal body weight.

- *Alcohol*—There is substantial evidence that alcohol consumption is associated with increased breast cancer risk. However, it is uncertain whether reducing alcohol consumption would decrease breast cancer risk.

- *Dietary Fat*—Although early studies suggested a possible association between a high-fat diet and increased breast cancer risk, more recent studies have been inconclusive. In the WHI, a low-fat diet did not help reduce breast cancer risk.

Chapter 21: Cancer Clusters

Defining Disease Clusters

A disease cluster is the occurrence of a greater than expected number of cases of a particular disease within a group of people, a geographic area, or a period of time. Clusters of diseases have concerned scientists for centuries. Some recent disease clusters include the initial cases of a rare type of pneumonia among homosexual men in the early 1980s that led to the identification of the human immunodeficiency virus (HIV) and acquired immunodeficiency syndrome (AIDS); the outbreak in 2003 of a respiratory illness, later identified as severe acute respiratory syndrome (SARS), caused by a previously unrecognized virus; and periodic outbreaks of food poisoning caused by eating food contaminated with bacteria.

Cancer clusters may be suspected when people report that several family members, friends, neighbors, or coworkers have been diagnosed with the same or related cancer(s). In the 1960s, one of the best known cancer clusters emerged, involving many cases of mesothelioma (a rare cancer of the lining of the chest and abdomen). Researchers traced the development of mesothelioma to exposure to asbestos, a fibrous mineral that was used heavily in shipbuilding during World War II and has also been used in manufacturing industrial and consumer products. Working with asbestos is the major risk factor (something that may increase the chance of developing a disease) for mesothelioma.

Facts About Cancer

Some concepts about cancer can be helpful when trying to understand suspected cancer clusters:

- Cancer is the uncontrolled growth and spread of abnormal cells anywhere in the body. However, cancer is not just one disease; it is actually an umbrella term for at least 100 different but related diseases.
- Each type of cancer has certain known and/or suspected risk factors associated with it.
- Cancer is not caused by injuries, nor is it contagious. It cannot be passed from one person to another like a cold or flu virus.
- Cancer is almost always caused by a combination of factors that interact in ways that are not yet fully understood.

- Carcinogenesis (the process by which normal cells are transformed into cancer cells) involves a series of changes within cells that usually occur over many years. More than 10 years can go by between the exposure to a carcinogen (any substance that causes cancer) and a diagnosis of cancer, which makes it difficult to pinpoint the cause of that cancer.

- Cancer is more likely to occur as people get older; because people are living longer, more cases of cancer can be expected in the future. This increased life expectancy may create the impression that cancer is becoming much more common, even though an increase in the number of cases of cancer is related in large part to the growing number of elderly people in the population.

- Some racial and ethnic groups have higher rates of cancer than other racial and ethnic groups. Such differences may be due to multiple factors, such as late stage of disease at diagnosis, barriers to health care access, history of other diseases, biologic and genetic differences, health behaviors, and other risk factors.

- Cancer, in general, is common. More than 17 million new cases of cancer have been diagnosed since 1990.

Facts About Cancer Clusters

Reported disease clusters of any kind, including suspected cancer clusters, are investigated by epidemiologists (scientists who study the frequency, distribution, causes, and control of diseases in populations). Epidemiologists use their knowledge of diseases, environmental science, lifestyle factors, and biostatistics to try to determine whether a suspected cluster represents a true excess of cancer cases.

Epidemiologists have identified certain circumstances that may lead them to suspect a potential common source or cause of cancer among people thought to be part of a cancer cluster. A suspected cancer cluster is more likely to be a true cluster, rather than a coincidence, if it involves one or more of the following factors:

- A large number of cases of one type of cancer, rather than several different types.
- A rare type of cancer, rather than common types.

- An increased number of cases of a certain type of cancer in an age group that is not usually affected by that type of cancer.

Before epidemiologists can assess a suspected cancer cluster accurately, they must determine whether the type of cancer involved is a primary (original) cancer or a cancer that has metastasized (spread from another organ). This is important to know because scientists consider only the primary cancer when they investigate a possible cancer cluster. Epidemiologists also try to establish whether the suspected exposure has the potential to cause the reported cancer, based on what is known about that cancer's likely causes and about the cancer-causing potential of the exposure.

After developing a case definition (the guidelines that determine whether the cases being investigated are related to the cluster), epidemiologists must identify the time period of concern and the population at risk. They then calculate the expected number of cases and compare that number with the observed number of cases.

Epidemiologists must show that the number of cancer cases that have occurred is significantly greater than the expected number of cases, given the age, gender, and racial distribution of the group of people at risk of developing the disease.

Epidemiologists must also determine if the cancer cases could have occurred by chance. They often test for "statistical significance," which is a mathematical measure of the difference between groups. The difference is said to be statistically significant if it is greater than what would be expected to happen by chance alone. In common practice, a statistically significant finding means that the probability that the observed number of cases could have happened by chance alone is 5 percent or less. For instance, if one examines the number of cancer cases in 100 neighborhoods, and cancer cases are occurring by chance alone, one should expect to find about five neighborhoods with a statistically significant elevation in the number of cancer cases. In other words, some amount of clustering within the same family or neighborhood may occur simply by chance.

Accurately defining the group of people who should be considered "at risk" is important when investigating a possible cancer cluster. One of the greatest problems in defining clusters is the tendency to expand the geographic borders of the cluster to include additional cases of the suspected disease as they are discovered. The tendency to define the borders of a cluster on the basis of where known cases are located, rather than to first define the population and geographic area and then determine if the number of cancers is excessive, creates many "clusters" that are not real.

Epidemiologists must also consider that a confirmed cancer cluster may not be the result of any single, external cause or hazard. A cancer cluster could be the result of chance, an error in the calculation of the expected number of cancer cases, or differences in the case definition between observed and expected cases. Moreover, because people change where they live from time to time, it can be difficult for epidemiologists to identify previous exposures and find the medical records that are needed to determine the kind of cancer a person had—or if it was cancer at all.

Because a variety of factors often work together to create the appearance of a cluster where nothing abnormal is occurring, most reports of suspected cancer clusters are not shown to be true clusters. Many reported clusters do not include enough cases for epidemiologists to arrive at any conclusions. Sometimes, even when a suspected cluster has enough cases for study, a greater than expected number of cases cannot be demonstrated. Other times, epidemiologists find a true excess of cases, but they cannot find an explanation for it. For example, a suspected carcinogen may cause cancer only under certain circumstances, making its impact difficult to detect.

Genetics and Environment

Because most cancers are thought to be caused by a combination of factors related to genetics and environment (including behavior and lifestyle), studies of suspected cancer clusters usually focus on these two issues. Genetic factors are inherited, that is, passed from parents to children. However, establishing a genetic-environmental interaction (significant and valid evidence that a specific genetic factor leads to an increased chance that a particular environmental exposure will result in cancer) requires studies of large populations over long periods of time. Researchers are just beginning to learn about the roles genetics and environmental exposures play in carcinogenesis. Some of their discoveries are outlined below:

Genetics

- All cancers develop because of genetic alterations of one kind or another. An alteration is a change or mutation in the physical structure of a gene that interferes with the gene's normal functions.

- Some genetic alterations that increase the risk of cancer are present at birth in the genes of all cells in the body, including reproductive cells. These changes, which are called germline mutations, can be passed from parent to child. This type of alteration is known as an inherited susceptibility; most cancers are not due to an inherited susceptibility.

- Most cancers result from genetic changes that occur after birth during one's lifetime. Genetic changes can occur in any cell that divides. These genetic changes are called somatic alterations.

- Familial cancer clusters (cancer that occurs in families more often than would be expected by chance) have been reported for many types of cancer. Because cancer is a common disease, it is not unusual for several cases to occur within a family. Familial cancer clusters are sometimes linked to inherited susceptibility, but environmental factors and chance may also be involved.

- Having an inherited susceptibility for a type of cancer does not necessarily mean that the individual will be diagnosed with the cancer; it means the chance of developing cancer increases if other factors that promote the development of cancer are present or are encountered later.

Environment

- The term environment includes not only air, water, and soil, but also substances and conditions in the home and workplace. It also includes diet; the use of tobacco, alcohol, or drugs; exposure to chemicals; and exposure to sunlight and other forms of radiation.

- People are exposed to a variety of environmental factors for varying lengths of time, and these factors interact in ways that are still not fully understood. Further, individuals have varying levels of susceptibility to these factors.

- Hazardous substances are often found in higher levels in the workplace than in the general environment. For this reason, some workers may have greater and longer exposures to such substances than the general population. Findings of higher than expected numbers of cancer cases among workers in particular occupations or industries provide important leads regarding causes of cancer among the general public. In fact, occupational studies (studies of specific groups of workers) have identified many specific cancer-causing substances and have provided the motivation to find ways to reduce or eliminate exposures in the workplace and elsewhere.

Chapter 22: Helicobacter pylori and Cancer

- Helicobacter pylori (H. pylori) is a type of bacterium that is found in the stomach of about two-thirds of the world's population.
- H. pylori infection is a major cause of gastric (stomach) cancer and is associated with an increased risk of gastric mucosa-associated lymphoid tissue (MALT) lymphoma.
- H. pylori infection may be associated with a decreased risk of some other cancers, including esophageal adenocarcinoma.

What is *Helicobacter pylori*?

Helicobacter pylori, or H. pylori, is a spiral-shaped bacterium that grows in the mucus layer that coats the inside of the human stomach.

To survive in the harsh, acidic environment of the stomach, H. pylori secretes an enzyme called urease, which converts the chemical urea to ammonia. The production of ammonia around H. pylori neutralizes the acidity of the stomach, making it more hospitable for the bacterium. In addition, the helical shape of H. pylori allows it to burrow into the mucus layer, which is less acidic than the inside space, or lumen, of the stomach. H. pylori can also attach to the cells that line the inner surface of the stomach.

Although immune cells that normally recognize and attack invading bacteria accumulate near sites of H. pylori infection, they are unable to reach the stomach lining. In addition, H. pylori has developed ways of interfering with local immune responses, making them ineffective in eliminating the bacteria.

H. pylori has coexisted with humans for many thousands of years and infection with the bacterium is common. The Centers for Disease Control and Prevention (CDC) estimates that approximately two-thirds of the world's population harbors the bacterium, with infection rates much higher in developing countries than in developed nations. Although H. pylori infection does not cause illness in most infected people, it is a major risk factor for peptic ulcer disease and is responsible for the majority of ulcers of the stomach and upper small intestine. The National Institute of Diabetes and Digestive and Kidney Diseases has more information about H. pylori and peptic ulcer disease.

In 1994, the International Agency for Research on Cancer classified H. pylori as a carcinogen, or cancer-causing agent, in humans, despite conflicting results at the time.

Since then, colonization of the stomach with H. pylori has been increasingly accepted as an important cause of stomach cancer and of gastric mucosa-associated lymphoid tissue (MALT) lymphoma. Infection with the bacteria is also associated with a reduced risk of esophageal adenocarcinoma.

Spread of H. pylori is thought to occur through contaminated food and water or through direct mouth-to-mouth contact. In most populations, the bacterium is first acquired during childhood. Children living in crowded conditions and with a lower socioeconomic status are more likely to become infected.

What is gastric cancer?

Gastric cancer, or cancer of the stomach, was once considered a single entity. Now, scientists divide this cancer into two main classes: gastric cardia cancer (cancer of the top inch of the stomach, where it meets the esophagus) and non-cardia gastric cancer (cancer in all other areas of the stomach).

In each of the last 5 years in the United States, approximately 21,000 new cases of gastric cancer were diagnosed and more than 10,000 deaths were caused by the disease. Gastric cancer is the second most common cause of cancer-related deaths in the world, killing approximately 738,000 people in 2008. Gastric cancer is less common in the United States and other Western countries than in countries in Asia and South America. Overall, gastric cancer incidence rates are decreasing. However, this decline is mainly in the rates of non-cardia gastric cancer. Gastric cardia cancer, which was once very uncommon, now constitutes nearly half of all stomach cancers among white males in the United States. Infection with H. pylori is the primary identified cause of gastric cancer. Other factors that increase the risk for gastric cancer include chronic gastritis; older age; male sex; a diet high in salted, smoked, or poorly preserved foods and low in fruits and vegetables; tobacco smoking; pernicious anemia; a history of stomach surgery for benign conditions; and a family history of stomach cancer.

What evidence shows that *H. pylori* infection causes gastric cancer?

Epidemiology studies have shown that individuals infected with H. pylori have an increased risk of gastric adenocarcinoma. In 2001, a combined analysis of 12 studies of H. pylori and gastric cancer estimated that the risk of adenocarcinoma in non-cardia regions of the stomach was nearly six times higher for H. pylori-infected people than for uninfected people.

Evidence for an association comes mainly from prospective cohort studies such as the Alpha-Tocopherol, Beta-Carotene (ATBC) Cancer Prevention Study in Finland, which involved nearly 30,000 male smokers who were aged 50 to 69 years at study enrollment. This study was designed to determine whether daily supplementation with alpha-tocopherol, beta-carotene, or both would reduce the number of lung or other cancers. H. pylori infection status was determined by analyzing blood samples obtained from each study participant at the time of enrollment in the study to see if they contained antibodies to the bacterium. Participants were enrolled during 1985 through 1988 and followed through 1999. Comparing subjects who developed gastric cancer with noncancer control subjects, the researchers found that H. pylori-infected individuals had a nearly eightfold increased risk for non-cardia gastric cancer.

Can treatment to eradicate *H. pylori* infection reduce gastric cancer rates?

Only two clinical trials have been conducted to determine whether eradicating H. pylori infection with antimicrobial therapy will reduce the incidence of gastric cancer. The total number of gastric cancers that developed in these studies was too small to make definitive statements. However, a meta-analysis of six randomized trials suggested that eradication may lead to a modest reduction in gastric cancer risk, because study participants were less likely to have precancerous lesions worsen if their H. pylori infections were eliminated.

What is gastric mucosa-associated lymphoid tissue (MALT) lymphoma, and what is the evidence that it can be caused by *H. pylori* infection?

Gastric MALT lymphoma is a rare type of non-Hodgkin lymphoma that is characterized by the slow multiplication of B lymphocytes, a type of immune cell, in the stomach lining. This cancer represents approximately 12 percent of the extranodal (outside of lymph nodes) non-Hodgkin lymphoma that occurs among men and approximately 18 percent of extranodal non-Hodgkin lymphoma among women. During the period 1999–2003, the annual incidence of gastric MALT lymphoma in the United States was about one case for every 100,000 persons in the population.

Normally, the lining of the stomach lacks lymphoid (immune system) tissue, but development of this tissue is often stimulated in response to colonization of the lining by H. pylori. Only in rare cases does this tissue give rise to MALT lymphoma. However, nearly all patients with gastric MALT lymphoma show signs of H. pylori infection, and the risk of developing this tumor is more than six times higher in infected people than in uninfected people.

What is the evidence that *H. pylori* infection may reduce the risk of some cancers?

The ATBC cohort study revealed that the risk of gastric cardia cancer among H. pylori-infected individuals was about one-third of that among uninfected individuals. Several other studies have also detected an inverse relationship between H. pylori infection and gastric cardia cancer, although the evidence is not entirely consistent. The possibility of an inverse relationship between the bacterium and gastric cardia cancer is supported by the corresponding decrease in H. pylori infection rates in Western countries during the past century—the result of improved hygiene and widespread antibiotic use—and the increase in rates of gastric cardia cancer in these same regions.

Similar epidemiologic evidence suggests that H. pylori infection may be associated with a lower risk of esophageal adenocarcinoma. For example, a large case-control study in Sweden showed that the risk of esophageal adenocarcinoma in H. pylori-infected individuals was one-third that of uninfected individuals. A meta-analysis of 13 studies, including the Swedish study, found a 45 percent reduction in risk of esophageal adenocarcinoma with H. pylori infection. Moreover, as with gastric cardia cancer, dramatic increases in esophageal adenocarcinoma rates in several Western countries parallel the declines in H. pylori infection rates.

How might *H. pylori* infection decrease the risk of some cancers while increasing the risk of other cancers?

Although it is not known for certain how H. pylori infection increases the risk of gastric cancer, some researchers speculate that the long-term presence of an inflammatory response predisposes cells in the stomach lining to become cancerous. This idea is supported by the finding that increased expression of a single cytokine (interleukin-1-beta) in the stomach of transgenic mice causes sporadic gastric inflammation and cancer. The increased cell turnover resulting from ongoing cellular damage could increase the likelihood that cells will develop harmful mutations.

One hypothesis that may explain reduced risks of gastric cardia and esophageal adenocarcinoma in H. pylori-infected individuals relates to the decline in stomach acidity that is often seen after decades of H. pylori colonization. This decline would reduce acid reflux into the esophagus, a major risk factor for adenocarcinomas affecting the upper stomach and esophagus.

What is *cagA*-positive *H. pylori* and how does it affect the risk of gastric and esophageal cancers?

Some H. pylori bacteria use a needle-like appendage to inject a toxin produced by a gene called cytotoxin-associated gene A (cagA) into the junctions where cells of the stomach lining meet. This toxin (known as CagA) alters the structure of stomach cells and allows the bacteria to attach to them more easily. Long-term exposure to the toxin causes chronic inflammation. However, not all strains of H. pylori carry the cagA gene; those that do are classified as cagA-positive.

Epidemiologic evidence suggests that infection with cagA-positive strains is especially associated with an increased risk of non-cardia gastric cancer and with reduced risks of gastric cardia cancer and esophageal adenocarcinoma. For example, a meta-analysis of 16 case-control studies conducted around the world showed that individuals infected with cagA-positive H. pylori had twice the risk of non-cardia gastric cancer than individuals infected with cagA-negative H. pylori. Conversely, a case-control study conducted in Sweden found that people infected with cagA-positive H. pylori had a statistically significantly reduced risk of esophageal adenocarcinoma. Similarly, another case-control study conducted in the United States found that infection with cagA-positive H. pylori was associated with a reduced risk of esophageal adenocarcinoma and gastric cardia cancer combined, but that infection with cagA-negative strains was not associated with risk. Recent research has suggested a potential mechanism by which CagA could contribute to gastric carcinogenesis. In three studies, infection with CagA-positive H. pylori was associated with inactivation of tumor suppressor proteins, including p53.

Is *H. pylori* infection associated with any other cancer?

A possible association between H. pylori infection and pancreatic cancer was suggested by several small epidemiology studies that found an increased risk of pancreatic cancer among patients who had been treated with surgery for peptic ulcer disease up to 20 years earlier. Furthermore, in the ATBC cohort study, individuals infected with H. pylori at the time of study enrollment were approximately twice as likely to develop pancreatic cancer as those without the infection.

However, this association between H. pylori infection and pancreatic cancer was not confirmed in another study that involved 128,992 adults. When the participants who developed pancreatic cancer were compared with control subjects, no evidence was found that individuals infected with H. pylori at study enrollment were more likely to develop pancreatic cancer than those who were not infected.

The relationship between H. pylori and colorectal cancer has also been studied. In a nested case-control study of men in the ATBC cancer prevention clinical trial, researchers found no evidence of H. pylori being a risk factor for colorectal adenocarcinoma.

Chapter 23: HIV Infection and Cancer Risk

Do people infected with human immunodeficiency virus (HIV) have an increased risk of cancer?

Yes. People infected with HIV have a substantially higher risk of some types of cancer compared with uninfected people of the same age. Three of these cancers are known as "acquired immunodeficiency syndrome (AIDS)-defining cancers" or "AIDS-defining malignancies": Kaposi sarcoma, non-Hodgkin lymphoma, and cervical cancer. A diagnosis of any one of these cancers marks the point at which HIV infection has progressed to AIDS.

People infected with HIV are several thousand times more likely than uninfected people to be diagnosed with Kaposi sarcoma, at least 70 times more likely to be diagnosed with non-Hodgkin lymphoma, and, among women, at least 5 times more likely to be diagnosed with cervical cancer.

In addition, people infected with HIV are at higher risk of several other types of cancer. These other malignancies include anal, liver, and lung cancer, and Hodgkin lymphoma.

People infected with HIV are at least 25 times more likely to be diagnosed with anal cancer than uninfected people, 5 times as likely to be diagnosed with liver cancer, 3 times as likely to be diagnosed with lung cancer, and at least 10 times more likely to be diagnosed with Hodgkin lymphoma.

People infected with HIV do not have increased risks of breast, colorectal, prostate, or many other common types of cancer. Screening for these cancers in HIV-infected people should follow current guidelines for the general population.

Why do people infected with HIV have a higher risk of cancer?

Infection with HIV weakens the immune system and reduces the body's ability to fight infections that may lead to cancer. Many people infected with HIV are also infected with other viruses that cause certain cancers. The following are the most important of these cancer-related viruses:

- Human herpesvirus 8 (HHV-8), also known as Kaposi sarcoma-associated herpesvirus (KSHV), is the cause of Kaposi sarcoma.
- Epstein Barr virus (EBV) causes some subtypes of non-Hodgkin and Hodgkin lymphoma.
- Human papillomavirus (HPV) causes cervical cancer and some types of anal, penile, vaginal, vulvar, and head and neck cancer.

- Hepatitis B virus (HBV) and hepatitis C virus (HCV) both can cause liver cancer.

Infection with most of these viruses is more common among people infected with HIV than among uninfected people.

In addition, the prevalence of some traditional risk factors for cancer, especially smoking (a known cause of lung cancer) and heavy alcohol use (which can increase the risk of liver cancer), is higher among people infected with HIV.

Has the introduction of antiretroviral therapy changed the cancer risk of people infected with HIV?

The introduction of highly active antiretroviral therapy (HAART) in the mid-1990s greatly reduced the incidence of Kaposi sarcoma and non-Hodgkin lymphoma among people infected with HIV. HAART lowers the amount of HIV circulating in the blood, thereby allowing partial restoration of immune system function.

Although lower than before, the risk of these two cancers is still much higher among people infected with HIV than among people in the general population. This persistently high risk may be due, at least in part, to the fact that immune system function remains substantially impaired in people treated with HAART. In addition, over time HIV can develop resistance to the drugs used in HAART. Many people infected with HIV have had difficulty in accessing medical care or taking their medication as prescribed. Although HAART has led to reductions in the incidence of Kaposi sarcoma and non-Hodgkin lymphoma among HIV-infected individuals, it has not reduced the incidence of cervical cancer, which has essentially remained unchanged. Moreover, the incidence of several other cancers, particularly Hodgkin lymphoma and anal cancer, has been increasing among HIV-infected individuals since the introduction of HAART. The influence of HAART on the risk of these other cancer types is not well understood. As HAART has reduced the number of deaths from AIDS, the HIV-infected population has grown in size and become older. The fastest growing proportion of HIV-infected individuals is the over-40 age group. These individuals are now developing cancers common in older age. In 2003, the proportion of these other cancers exceeded the number of AIDS-defining malignancies. However, HIV-infected people do not develop most cancers at a younger age than is typically seen in the general population

What can people infected with HIV do to reduce their risk of cancer or to find cancer early?

Taking HAART as indicated based on current HIV treatment guidelines lowers the risk of Kaposi sarcoma and non-Hodgkin lymphoma and increases overall survival. The risk of lung cancer can be reduced by quitting smoking. Because HIV-infected people have a higher risk of lung cancer, it is especially important that they do not smoke.

The higher incidence of liver cancer among HIV-infected people appears to be related to more frequent infection with hepatitis virus (particularly HCV) and alcohol abuse or dependence than among uninfected people. Therefore, HIV-infected individuals should know their hepatitis status. If blood tests show that they have previously been infected with HBV or HCV, they should consider reducing their alcohol consumption.

In addition, if they currently have viral hepatitis, they should discuss with their health care provider whether HBV- or HCV-suppressing therapy is an option for them. Some drugs may be used for both HBV-suppressing therapy and HAART.

Because HIV-infected women have a higher risk of cervical cancer, it is important that they be screened regularly for this disease. Studies have suggested that Pap test abnormalities are more common among HIV-infected women and that HPV DNA tests may not be as effective as Pap tests in screening these women for cervical cancer. Some researchers recommend anal Pap test screening to detect and treat early lesions before they progress to anal cancer. This type of screening may be most beneficial for men who have had sexual intercourse with other men. HIV-infected patients should discuss such screening with their medical providers.

Chapter 24: Obesity and Cancer Risk

- During the past several decades, the percentage of overweight and obese adults and children has increased markedly.
- Obesity is associated with increased risks of cancers of the esophagus, breast (postmenopausal), endometrium (the lining of the uterus), colon and rectum, kidney, pancreas, thyroid, gallbladder, and possibly other cancer types.
- Obese people are also at higher risk of coronary heart disease, stroke, high blood pressure, diabetes, and a number of other chronic diseases.

What is obesity?

Obesity is a condition in which a person has an abnormally high and unhealthy proportion of body fat.

To measure obesity, researchers commonly use a scale known as the body mass index (BMI). BMI is calculated by dividing a person's weight (in kilograms) by their height (in meters) squared. BMI provides a more accurate measure of obesity or being overweight than weight alone.

Guidelines established by the National Institutes of Health (NIH) place adults age 20 and older into the following categories based on their BMI:

BMI	BMI Categories
Below 18.5	Underweight
18.5 to 24.9	Normal
25.0 to 29.9	Overweight
30.0 and above	Obese

The National Heart Lung and Blood Institute provides a BMI calculator .

For children and adolescents (less than 20 years of age), overweight and obesity are based on the Centers for Disease Control and Prevention's (CDC) BMI-for-age growth charts:

BMI	BMI Categories
BMI-for-age at or above sex-specific 85th percentile, but less than 95th percentile	Overweight
BMI-for-age at or above sex-specific 95th percentile	Obese

Compared with people of normal weight, those who are overweight or obese are at greater risk for many diseases, including diabetes, high blood pressure, cardiovascular diseases, stroke, and certain cancers.

How common is overweight or obesity?

Results from the 2007-2008 National Health and Nutrition Examination Survey (NHANES) show that 68 percent of U.S. adults age 20 years and older are overweight or obese. In 1988-1994, by contrast, only 56 percent of adults age 20 and older were overweight or obese.

In addition, the percentage of children who are overweight or obese has also increased. Among children and teens ages 2 to 19, 17 percent are estimated to be obese, based on the 2007–2008 survey. In 1988–1994, that figure was only 10 percent.

What is known about the relationship between obesity and cancer?

Obesity is associated with increased risks of the following cancer types, and possibly others as well:

- Esophagus
- Pancreas
- Colon and rectum

- Breast (after menopause)
- Endometrium (lining of the uterus)
- Kidney
- Thyroid
- Gallbladder

One study, using NCI Surveillance, Epidemiology, and End Results (SEER) data, estimated that in 2007 in the United States, about 34,000 new cases of cancer in men (4 percent) and 50,500 in women (7 percent) were due to obesity. The percentage of cases attributed to obesity varied widely for different cancer types but was as high as 40 percent for some cancers, particularly endometrial cancer and esophageal adenocarcinoma.

A projection of the future health and economic burden of obesity in 2030 estimated that continuation of existing trends in obesity will lead to about 500,000 additional cases of cancer in the United States by 2030. This analysis also found that if every adult reduced their BMI by 1 percent, which would be equivalent to a weight loss of roughly 1 kg (or 2.2 lbs) for an adult of average weight, this would prevent the increase in the number of cancer cases and actually result in the avoidance of about 100,000 new cases of cancer.

Several possible mechanisms have been suggested to explain the association of obesity with increased risk of certain cancers:

- Fat tissue produces excess amounts of estrogen, high levels of which have been associated with the risk of breast, endometrial, and some other cancers.

- Obese people often have increased levels of insulin and insulin-like growth factor-1 (IGF-1) in their blood (a condition known as hyperinsulinemia or insulin resistance), which may promote the development of certain tumors.

- Fat cells produce hormones, called adipokines, that may stimulate or inhibit cell growth. For example, leptin, which is more abundant in obese people, seems to promote cell proliferation, whereas adiponectin, which is less abundant in obese people, may have antiproliferative effects.

- Fat cells may also have direct and indirect effects on other tumor growth regulators, including mammalian target of rapamycin (mTOR) and AMP-activated protein kinase.

- Obese people often have chronic low-level, or "subacute," inflammation, which has been associated with increased cancer risk.

Other possible mechanisms include altered immune responses, effects on the nuclear factor kappa beta system, and oxidative stress.

What is known about the relationship between obesity and breast cancer?

Many studies have shown that overweight and obesity are associated with a modest increase in risk of postmenopausal breast cancer. This higher risk is seen mainly in women who have never used menopausal hormone therapy (MHT) and for tumors that express both estrogen and progesterone receptors.

Overweight and obesity have, by contrast, been found to be associated with a reduced risk of premenopausal breast cancer in some studies.

The relationship between obesity and breast cancer may be affected by the stage of life in which a woman gains weight and becomes obese. Epidemiologists are actively working to address this question. Weight gain during adult life, most often from about age 18 to between the ages of 50 and 60, has been consistently associated with risk of breast cancer after menopause.

The increased risk of postmenopausal breast cancer is thought to be due to increased levels of estrogen in obese women. After menopause, when the ovaries stop producing hormones, fat tissue becomes the most important source of estrogen. Because obese women have more fat tissue, their estrogen levels are higher, potentially leading to more rapid growth of estrogen-responsive breast tumors.

The relationship between obesity and breast cancer risk may also vary by race and ethnicity. There is limited evidence that the risk associated with overweight and obesity may be less among African American and Hispanic women than among white women.

What is known about the relationship between obesity and endometrial cancer?

Overweight and obesity have been consistently associated with endometrial cancer, which is cancer of the lining of the uterus. Obese and overweight women have two to four times the risk of developing this disease than women of a normal weight, regardless of menopausal status. Many studies have also found that the risk of endometrial cancer increases with increasing weight gain in adulthood, particularly among women who have never used MHT. Although it has not yet been determined why obesity is a risk factor for endometrial cancer, some evidence points to a role for diabetes, possibly in combination with low levels of physical activity. High levels of estrogen produced by fat tissue are also likely to play a role.

What is known about the relationship between obesity and colorectal cancer?

Among men, a higher BMI is strongly associated with increased risk of colorectal cancer. The distribution of body fat appears to be an important factor, with abdominal obesity, which can be measured by waist circumference, showing the strongest association with colon cancer risk. An association between BMI and waist circumference with colon cancer risk is also seen in women, but it is weaker. Use of MHT may modify the association in postmenopausal women.

A number of mechanisms have been proposed to account for the association of obesity with increased colon cancer risk. One hypothesis is that high levels of insulin or insulin-related growth factors in obese people may promote colon cancer development.

High BMI is also associated with rectal cancer risk, but the increase in risk is more modest.

What is known about the relationship between obesity and kidney cancer?

Obesity has been consistently associated with renal cell cancer, which is the most common form of kidney cancer, in both men and women. The mechanisms by which obesity may increase renal cell cancer risk are not well understood. High blood pressure is a known risk factor for renal cell cancer, but the relationship between obesity and kidney cancer is independent of blood pressure status. High levels of insulin may play a role in the development of the disease.

What is known about the relationship between obesity and esophageal cancer?

Overweight and obese people are about twice as likely as people of healthy weight to develop a type of esophageal cancer called esophageal adenocarcinoma. Most studies have observed no increased risk, or even a decline in risk, with obesity for the other major type of esophageal cancer, squamous cell cancer.

The mechanisms by which obesity may increase risk of esophageal adenocarcinoma are not well understood. However, overweight and obese people are more likely than people of normal weight to have a history of gastroesophageal reflux disease or Barrett esophagus, which are associated with an increased risk of esophageal adenocarcinoma. It is possible that obesity exacerbates the esophageal inflammation that is associated with these conditions.

What is known about the relationship between obesity and pancreatic cancer?

Many studies have reported a slight increase in risk of pancreatic cancer among overweight and obese individuals. Waist circumference may be a particularly important factor in the association of overweight and obesity with pancreatic cancer.

What is known about the relationship between obesity and thyroid cancer?

Increasing weight has been found to be associated with an increase in the risk of thyroid cancer. It is unclear what the mechanism might be.

What is known about the relationship between obesity and gallbladder cancer?

The risk of gallbladder cancer increases with increasing BMI. The increase in risk may be due to the higher frequency of gallstones, a strong risk factor for gallbladder cancer, in obese individuals

What is known about the relationship between obesity and other cancers?

The relationship between obesity and prostate cancer has been studied extensively. The results of individual studies do not suggest a consistent association between obesity and prostate cancer. However, when the data from multiple studies are pooled, analyses show that obesity may be associated with a very slight increase in the risk of prostate cancer.

In addition, several studies have found that obese men have a higher risk of aggressive prostate cancer than men of healthy weight. Generally, risk of prostate cancer has been linked to levels of certain hormones and growth factors, especially IGF-1.

Some studies have shown a weak association between increasing BMI and risk of ovarian cancer, especially in premenopausal women, although other studies have not found an association. As with some other cancers, an association between ovarian cancer and obesity may reflect increased levels of estrogens.

Some evidence links obesity to liver cancer and to some types of lymphoma and leukemia, but additional studies are needed to confirm these associations.

Does avoiding weight gain or losing weight decrease the risk of cancer?

The most conclusive way to test whether avoiding weight gain or losing weight will decrease the risk of cancer is through a controlled clinical trial. A number of NIH-funded weight loss trials have demonstrated that people can lose weight and that losing weight reduces their risk of developing chronic diseases, such as diabetes, while improving their risk factors for cardiovascular disease. However, previous trials and the results of an NCI workshop have demonstrated that it would not be feasible to conduct a weight loss trial of cancer prevention. The reason is that the effect of weight loss on the prevention of other chronic diseases would be demonstrated—and the trial consequently stopped so that the public could be informed of the benefits—before the effect on the prevention of cancer would become evident.

Therefore, most data about whether losing weight or avoiding weight gain prevents cancer come mainly from cohort and case-control studies. Data from these types of studies, called observational studies, can be difficult to interpret because people who lose weight or avoid weight gain may be different in other ways from people who do not, just as obese people may differ from lean people in other ways than BMI. That is, it is possible that these other differences explain their different cancer risk.

Nevertheless, many observational studies have shown that people who have a lower weight gain during adulthood have a lower risk of:

- Colon cancer
- Breast cancer (after menopause)
- Endometrial cancer

A more limited number of observational studies have examined the relationship between weight loss and cancer risk, and a few have found decreased risks of breast cancer and colon cancer among people who have lost weight. However, most of these studies have not been able to evaluate whether the weight loss was intentional or related to underlying health problems.

Stronger evidence comes from studies of patients who have undergone bariatric surgery to lose weight. Obese people who have bariatric surgery appear to have lower rates of obesity-related cancers than obese people who did not have bariatric surgery. It is important to note that whereas most lifestyle weight loss interventions result in weight losses of 7-10 percent of body weight, weight loss from bariatric surgery combined with lifestyle changes generally results in weight loss of 30 percent.

Chapter 25: Psychological Stress and Cancer

- Psychological stress alone has not been found to cause cancer, but psychological stress that lasts a long time may affect a person's overall health and ability to cope with cancer.

- People who are better able to cope with stress have a better quality of life while they are being treated for cancer, but they do not necessarily live longer.

What is psychological stress?

Psychological stress describes what people feel when they are under mental, physical, or emotional pressure. Although it is normal to experience some psychological stress from time to time, people who experience high levels of psychological stress or who experience it repeatedly over a long period of time may develop health problems (mental and/or physical).

Stress can be caused both by daily responsibilities and routine events, as well as by more unusual events, such as a trauma or illness in oneself or a close family member. When people feel that they are unable to manage or control changes caused by cancer or normal life activities, they are in distress. Distress has become increasingly recognized as a factor that can reduce the quality of life of cancer patients. There is even some evidence that extreme distress is associated with poorer clinical outcomes. Clinical guidelines are available to help doctors and nurses assess levels of distress and help patients manage it.

How does the body respond during stress?

The body responds to physical, mental, or emotional pressure by releasing stress hormones (such as epinephrine and norepinephrine) that increase blood pressure, speed heart rate, and raise blood sugar levels. These changes help a person act with greater strength and speed to escape a perceived threat.

Research has shown that people who experience intense and long-term (i.e., chronic) stress can have digestive problems, fertility problems, urinary problems, and a weakened immune system. People who experience chronic stress are also more prone to viral infections such as the flu or common cold and to have headaches, sleep trouble, depression, and anxiety.

Can psychological stress cause cancer?

Although stress can cause a number of physical health problems, the evidence that it can cause cancer is weak. Some studies have indicated a link between various psychological factors and an increased risk of developing cancer, but others have not.

Apparent links between psychological stress and cancer could arise in several ways. For example, people under stress may develop certain behaviors, such as smoking, overeating, or drinking alcohol, which increase a person's risk for cancer. Or someone who has a relative with cancer may have a higher risk for cancer because of a shared inherited risk factor, not because of the stress induced by the family member's diagnosis.

How does psychological stress affect people who have cancer?

People who have cancer may find the physical, emotional, and social effects of the disease to be stressful. Those who attempt to manage their stress with risky behaviors such as smoking or drinking alcohol or who become more sedentary may have a poorer quality of life after cancer treatment. In contrast, people who are able to use effective coping strategies to deal with stress, such as relaxation and stress management techniques, have been shown to have lower levels of depression, anxiety, and symptoms related to the cancer and its treatment. However, there is no evidence that successful management of psychological stress improves cancer survival.

Evidence from experimental studies does suggest that psychological stress can affect a tumor's ability to grow and spread. For example, some studies have shown that when mice bearing human tumors were kept confined or isolated from other mice—conditions that increase stress—their tumors were more likely to grow and spread (metastasize). In one set of experiments, tumors transplanted into the mammary fat pads of mice had much higher rates of spread to the lungs and lymph nodes if the mice were chronically stressed than if the mice were not stressed. Studies in mice and in human cancer cells grown in the laboratory have found that the stress hormone norepinephrine, part of the body's fight-or-flight response system, may promote angiogenesis and metastasis.

In another study, women with triple-negative breast cancer who had been treated with neoadjuvant chemotherapy were asked about their use of beta blockers, which are medications that interfere with certain stress hormones, before and during chemotherapy. Women who reported using beta blockers had a better chance of surviving their cancer treatment without a relapse than women who did not report beta blocker use. There was no difference between the groups, however, in terms of overall survival.

Although there is still no strong evidence that stress directly affects cancer outcomes, some data do suggest that patients can develop a sense of helplessness or hopelessness when stress becomes overwhelming. This response is associated with higher rates of death, although the mechanism for this outcome is unclear. It may be that people who feel helpless or hopeless do not seek treatment when they become ill, give up prematurely on or fail to adhere to potentially helpful therapy, engage in risky behaviors such as drug use, or do not maintain a healthy lifestyle, resulting in premature death.

How can people who have cancer learn to cope with psychological stress?

Emotional and social support can help patients learn to cope with psychological stress. Such support can reduce levels of depression, anxiety, and disease- and treatment-related symptoms among patients. Approaches can include the following:

Training in relaxation, meditation, or stress management

- Counseling or talk therapy

- Cancer education sessions
- Social support in a group setting
- Medications for depression or anxiety
- Exercise

Some expert organizations recommend that all cancer patients be screened for distress early in the course of treatment. A number also recommend re-screening at critical points along the course of care. Health care providers can use a variety of screening tools, such as a distress scale or questionnaire, to gauge whether cancer patients need help managing their emotions or with other practical concerns. Patients who show moderate to severe distress are typically referred to appropriate resources, such as a clinical health psychologist, social worker, chaplain, or psychiatrist.

Other MedicalCenter.com
Publications

The Key Facts on Arthritis

The Key Facts on Breast Cancer

The Key Facts on Medicare

The Key Facts on Alzheimer's Disease

The Key Facts on Caring For Someone With

Alzheimer's Disease

The Key Facts on Cancer Series

All Titles Can Be Found at

www.Amazon.com

www.MedicalCenter.com